Combo Feeding

The Best of Both Worlds

By Sophia Felder, FNP, IBCLC

Introduction:

This book aims to integrate knowledge about lactation, infant feeding needs, infant feeding options, and mental health while caring for an infant. The knowledge shared here aims to help parents be empowered to make decisions that will work for their family. I understand that families need to make decisions that work for their lifestyle and preferences.

I firmly believe that knowledge is empowering. The more you know about a topic the more likely you are to succeed at doing it, and that means to feel good about the outcome and the journey. The steep learning curve that happens when you have a baby is currently too steep, especially for sleep deprived and vulnerable new parents. My aim in writing this book (and my others) is to flatten that learning curve and bring more education to the general public.

Nursing (or breastfeeding) and other infant feeding methods (like formula feeding) are often pitted against one another, but they do not have to be. Using data we have on biological optimization for maintaining lactation, we can bio-hack routines to be more sustainable. This can mean utilizing more than one feeding method at a time, otherwise known as combo-feeding. For the purpose of this book I am defining combo-feeding for an infant as utilizing multiple methods of getting the milk into the baby. That being said, pumping from the breast counts as feeding from the breast, therefore: pumping is breastfeeding. Combo-feeding may or may not include using formula, depending on milk supply, preferences, and goals. The knowledge I present will help parents go into managing feeding from a more informed space. The goal is that this will make room for a longer and more enjoyable lactation relationship. As it currently is, many parents wean before they planned due to lack of knowledge and support, as well as mounting frustration and stress. I believe combo-feeding can be a tool used to lessen the stress around infant feeding, and thus extend the lactation relationship.

This book serves to promote lactation relationship longevity through avoiding premature weaning that is based on lack of information or mismanagement of combination feeding strategies. My hope is to de-stigmatize combo feeding, make education on how to do so more accessible, and to make the feeding relationship less burdensome. Our nursing initiation rates are high, but continuation rates are low--and I am sure that part of this trend is lack of access to information and support for parents, but it doesn't have to be. I believe through education we can change that, and I hope this is what my books do.

About Me:

On a personal level, I have endured many challenges with lactation and infant feeding, and that has made me a more compassionate caregiver. I have had low supply, latch pain, thrush, tongue-tied babies, used nipple shields, pumped, bottle fed, taken medications, ingested herbs, used a supplemental nursing system, returned to work, dealt with harassment from coworkers, suffered blisters, endured infections, and managed clogged ducts. I have fought this fight four times. I have been there, done that, and bought the gadget.

I believe now that my breastfeeding problems were a gift to me. I have a heart of service and want to use my gifts to help others. I was especially gifted sympathy for those struggling with lactation. I deeply and personally know how it is such a vulnerable and special time, and how decisions around infant parenting can feel so heavy. I have felt the strong and innate drive to fight through challenges to just feed my child. I have felt the heartache of the self judgement that I was failing.

Professionally, I am a Family Nurse Practitioner and an Internationally Board-Certified Lactation Consultant. I have a Bachelor of Science in Psychology, Bachelor of Science in Nursing, and Master of Science in Nursing. I have worked in Maternal-Infant Health since 2012, and lactation support has always been part of my work, even when going into family practice as a provider in 2017. In 2018 I decided to make lactation medicine a focus of my practice. I believe that lactation relationships are an important aspect of health across the life-span, for both the lactating parent as well as the breastfed child.

I work full time as a Family Nurse Practitioner and have specialty knowledge in lactation. I see patients on the Olympic Peninsula in Washington State, and do some online consulting. In between work and parenting, I educate and connect with my readers and patients through my

Instagram found via @sophiafelder.fnp.ibclc. This is also where you can find information on how to book with me and purchase my other books.

For the greater part of the last decade of my life countless parents have expressed gratitude and appreciation for my candor and for educating them, so I figured I have something to offer on a larger scale. I have written, and am writing, other books to help educate parents about many of the challenges of lactation and modern parenting.

My general lactation education book "Can I talk you out of breastfeeding?" is a tongue-in-cheek title (so, not actually trying to talk you out of it) that has the educational material modern parents are actually craving. I was moved to write because I was repeatedly upset at hearing that parents felt unprepared for the realities of lactation (or infant feeding in general) and I seek to change the conversations we have around lactation and the mental health of new parents through my writing. I cover topics there that no other lactation book dares.

My book "Sleep Training the Breastfed Baby (or Not)" covers how sleep training might affect lactation, how to balance that, and many tips on getting rest even without sleep training. It is a topic that does not get as much coverage as it should in new parent education, and is an option many parents consider or are pressured to consider by well-meaning family and friends.

In general, I look at biological norms, biological data feedback, all the options, and then I look at the lactating parent and the infant as a whole and then again as separate units. My books are more than how to manuals, and give real and practical information. Mental health is at the forefront of my books and my aim is to empower parents to make the best personalized decisions for their families from an informed space. Resources for help are also included in each book.

In clinical practice and in my writing, I strive to provide evidence-based care, and sometimes all that I have is anecdotes. This is the current reality of the fast-paced world we live in. I do my best to balance it all, and use my best clinical judgement. Given my personal and professional background, I believe that I can help new parents. I have a passion to help, and to help parents through this time is my honor.

Disclaimer

This book is intended for educational and entertainment purposes only and does not replace medical advice following a thorough and detailed assessment by an appropriately credentialed provider. Reading this book does not establish a patient-provider relationship. The author disclaims any liability of outcomes based on the information provided in this book and expects all readers needing professional assistance to seek it in a timely and appropriate manner.

Chapters:

Why It Matters

I believe some context is important going into this journey, so we will explore that first. It can be challenging to deal with an abrupt change in lifestyle for a new and lactating parent. Additionally, these changes can affect our relationships with others. Cluster feeding, leaking, lack of sleep, growth spurts, teething, engorgement, and being the primary caretaker are just some of those challenges, and the challenges begin right away.

In a typical parent-child relationship, the parent who is lactating has a severe sleep deficit when they are waking frequently for night feedings. A completely normal part of taking care of a newborn is how the lack of sleep can affect a person. Parents do not get much sleep when they have a newborn, less if nursing does not go well. Babies are just very disruptive to sleep. In general, when we are exhausted, our physical and mental health is negatively impacted. Being exhausted just does not feel good.

Our exhaustion can make us edgy and negative. You may resent your baby when they wake more than usual at night. You also might resent your partner for sleeping through midnight feeds. Often when we are tired, we are more short-tempered and our emotions can be like a roller-coaster. During postpartum, the body and the soul are under a lot of pressure, meeting seemingly constant demands. Learning to adjust and grow with these big changes is really challenging, and its typical to have a hard time during this period.

What I just went over, obviously, can influence your relationships with others. Especially the people who live with us. Sleep deprivation can make that extra few minutes to spare seem like it should only be made available for a nap, and you would prioritize this over spending it being intimate with a partner or taking time to call a friend. The sheer exhaustion and workload of parenthood can make it hard to have time to get in the mood for partner intimacy, and exacerbate feelings of overstimulation, and being "touched-out." When we get a moment alone, we might crave to avoid stimulation of any kind. We lose time and energy to connect with our loved ones in the ways we used to.

Of utmost importance is the effect that infant parenting has on our mental health. Parents often expect to hold onto their joy and elation every moment of the postpartum experience. This can feel very jarring and incongruent with the reality of being exhausted and overwhelmed by a newborn. Then there is the self-shame for feeling this, which can lead to deeper and more consistent negative emotions. It is okay to not enjoy every moment or have moments of doubt and even negative feelings about having become a parent. At the same time, we may go in and out of feeling high on the love we have for our infant. When we are sleep deprived and struggling, this push and pull is normal. This risk can be true of all parents, of course, but especially optimistic, and high-achieving personalities.

If you are prone to mental illness or it runs in your family then it is a good idea to set up safety nets and support systems before you reach your postpartum period. Even parents with all the support in the world and all the sleep they crave can still develop postpartum mood disorders, because it is largely hormonally driven. It is always wise to be realistic and prepare for the possibilities, regardless of risk factors. Please do not anticipate that combo feeding will prevent or cure a mood disorder. I go much more in depth on lactation and mental health in my general lactation book, if you want more information this is a great resource.

In addition to our mental health and relationships with others, the information in this book is critical in helping parents reach their lactation goals and in feeling confident in their parenting decisions. Goals and expectations are usually in line with healthcare suggestions and guidelines, but parents lack the support and education needed to reach those goals. It shouldn't

be a surprise to new parents what biological norms are for their own bodies, or their infants'
bodies.

Combo-feeding is also typically a crucial component of meeting long term lactation goals
for parents who have to return to work outside the home. With the demands of work and home
life, the extra demands of pumping, and stress—often parents struggle to exclusively breastfeed
the recommended time frame. If we can extend lactation and access to breastmilk by reducing
the burden and introducing combination feeding, more people will meet their goals in terms of
length of time.

This leads me into saying that this topic also matters because of the potential effects on
health of both the lactating parent and infant. The longevity of the lactation relationship is more
important than the quantity. That is to say, length of time trumps amounts. The longer a female
lactates, the more she lowers risk of breast cancer, colorectal cancer, ovarian cancer, diabetes,
hypertension, dementia, and osteoporosis. The longer an infant or child receives human milk, the
more benefit to their thymus and immune system development. The longer they nurse, the more
benefit to their facial structural development. For these benefits we do not need to exclusively
provide breast milk, only to keep the relationship going for as long as possible (and desired).

There is also risk to the biological norms of the lactation process when we disrupt it. I
discuss supply building and regulation in detail, in order to explain the biology behind how
sometimes combo-feeding can go wrong and sabotage lactation. I also explain how for some
lactating parents there are ways around this, or at least how to minimize impacts. There are ways
to successfully balance the desire to combo-feed and share the load, while protecting lactation. It
can be a great relief to not be the sole provider of an infant's calories and hydration.

Formula, pumping, and bottles have given us many gifts in our modern life but relative to the history of humans it is only very recently that we have introduced these methods of infant feeding for the general population versus it being used by a select few. In many ways we are fighting thousands of years of what was normal for a majority of humans, to try to create a new normal. Historically, females used to always be surrounded by many other lactating females. Females had many babies over their entire life, from puberty to menopause, so most of them were lactating off and on for decades. Each subsequent pregnancy brought more mammary tissue growth, and thus more and more milk with each baby. People in general also lived in closer quarters. Villages were made of many tiny homes very close together, where we had much greater labor sharing of daily tasks. Having your friend or relative nurse your baby until your milk came in, or so you could get a break, was the norm. Having one person wet nurse several children so that others could focus on other jobs was the norm. Using a bit of milk from the goat or cow out back when you had low supply or had to be separated from the baby was also the norm. The human species is so flexible and resilient, and always has been!

Today, since we have pumping, bottles, and formula this gives us more options. We know that breastmilk from human parents is best for human babies; it is optimal. Yet many odds are stacked against the modern breastfeeding dyad. In many instances of parenting, beyond feeding, optimal is out of a realistic reach for many of us We do the best we can. We live in houses, separated from our neighbors, with our small family units. There is less collective community child-rearing. Many lactating parents work outside the home, adding additional pressure and complications to keeping a lactation relationship going. You do still have the option of using a wet nurse, but it is harder to accommodate that plan in our modern lifestyles and living arrangements, unless you live in a house with multiple lactating women. Additionally, you might be willing to spend time, money, and effort sourcing donor milk. If you want or need to use formula or other supplemental milk in your feeding routine, you can work to maximize (or at least maintain) your supply so that you can still meet your breastfeeding goals in terms of length of time spent nursing or lactating. If you have an abundant supply, you might be comfortable sacrificing some of it in order to make combo-feeding work for your family. Many parents combo feed and are able to make their long-term breastfeeding goals. Before the cultural big push to exclusively breast feed, many families happily did this without a second thought.

We also have to touch on that sometimes combo feeding is not a choice. We will explore this more in depth in a following chapter on low supply, but it definitely also demands to be mentioned here. Sometimes every effort can be made to boost supply without significant returns. We will explore in this book how to balance combo-feeding in that case, as well.

Whether by necessity or preference, combo feeding is the way a majority of parents choose to tackle infant feeding the first year of life. It is time education started reflecting the realities and preferences of modern parents.

Laying a Foundation

You start making milk (well, colostrum) while pregnant, and you might even leak! When your milk transitions from colostrum milk to mature milk a few days after the baby is born, you will likely experience engorgement. You can also develop mammary tissue anywhere along your "milk lines" which go from your armpits to your groin. Imagine the teats on other mammals such as cats and dogs to get a visual. Be prepared for possible swelling, extra nipples, leaking, or engorgement to possibly develop along the milk line.

Engorgement is a combination of the milk volume increasing, as well as water around the milk glands, this creates an uncomfortable tightness over the skin. This is often what others refer to when they say they felt their milk "come-in." Engorgement might be worse with each child but tends to resolve more quickly.

The edema in the chest that is part of the engorgement can be made worse when you are given a lot of fluids during labor and delivery. You will also notice a surge of edema in your hands and feet 1 to 3 days after delivery. The fluid needs displaced with lymph massage in the direction away from the breast, and will not always move or feel relieved when you try to remove milk. It seems contrary but drinking a lot of water helps stabilize the fluids in the body, and your body will release the extra fluids more readily if you are well-hydrated.

After engorgement resolves you will encounter more changes in your chest. The breasts will seem to soften and not feel full like they did in the early postpartum days. The first few weeks is a common time for parents to worry about milk seeming to dry up or go away. When this change couples up with cluster feeding many people quit, thinking they are not making enough milk. The mammae feeling full is actually a sign that they are not being drained well.

They should soften after this initial engorgement period, and feel softer still, after each feeding; feeling fuller only briefly right before the next feeding as they have refilled between feeds. After supply regulation the breasts continue to get flatter and have a less full feeling. This is because the mammae transition from being a storage warehouse, where milk is always ready to feed with some extra to spare, to a feed on demand factory where the milk is made and pulled out of the breast as the infant nurses and requests it. The mammae are never empty because the milk making is on a slow and continual process, so even if a baby nurses for a long time and the breast feels soft there is still milk coming, it is just at a slower rate than it was at the beginning of the feed. These changes are normal and expected, and you can check in with your lactation consultant about signs of low supply if the change worries you.

Many people who do not experience engorgement mistakenly assume that their milk never came in. It is possible if you have a baby that feeds very frequently and drains the mammae very well that you might avoid engorgement discomfort, and does not necessarily indicate a low supply. Many cases of low supply are only perceived low supply and not true medical low supply. Professional assessment is critical if you suspect insufficient milk supply or a dip in supply. Perceived low supply can be just as stressful, so we don't want to discount or dismiss it—you should always seek support from an IBCLC if you suspect it.

During the first few days of nursing you may also experience a new sensation in the breasts called a "let-down." We call it this because the cycle of hormones involves the brain sending hormones to the mammae, and then the breasts send the milk to the baby, all in a downward cascade. It is triggered by the suckling baby or pump, and this signals the brain to allow for the letdown to occur, so it is a feedback loop. The letdown involves the muscles around the milk ducts squeezing the milk out in faster and stronger gushes.

The letdown is a physical and hormonal occurrence. Many describe it as tingling, burning, or itching. Although, not everyone can feel their letdown in their chest. A let-down is often accompanied by a strong overwhelming tiredness, thirst, and hunger. This may be your only clue, along with hearing your baby gulping or swallowing, that a letdown as occurred.

The letdown is often pleasurable, but not always. The hormone oxytocin is largely responsible for this mechanism. Oxytocin is also responsible for contractions, orgasms, and bonding. When the newborn is nursing and the oxytocin surges it tells the body the baby is on the outside now, so it is time to shrink the uterus and make the milk. Not all people feel their letdown, so do not be discouraged if you cannot. Some also experience it in more unique ways, such as shoulder tension or a sudden negative emotional reaction. Typically, the early weeks will be when you feel the letdown the strongest. As your body adjusts the sensations might completely go away or at least be less intense. You are likely to stop feeling them when you nurse for a long time or are nursing your second or third child.

Now that you have some background on what to expect with bodily functions, we can get into laying the foundation for a good supply. Not removing the milk often enough or efficiently enough in the early postpartum days can be detrimental to supply. This is one of the risk factors that can cause chronic low supply. It is best to drain the breast as much as possible every 2-3 hours and to have no more than a single occurrence of a longer stretch than that every 24 hours. Generally, most people can get away with one stretch per day of 4 to 6 hours for rest without dramatic impact on over-all supply. The baby will still need to eat while we rest, until they are old enough and gaining weight well enough. Outside of that, expect 8 to 12 times in 24 hours of milk removal by hand-expressing, pumping, or nursing if you are aiming for establishing a full supply. This can be every 5 to 60 minutes when baby is cluster feeding, or every 2 to 3 hours for the longer stretches between feeds. Sometimes in the early weeks babies eat 12-16 times a day. Gradually as the milk supply is established your baby will stop cluster feeding so often and go for longer stretches between feeds more consistently. If the baby is not draining the breast, you will need to hand express or pump to do so. When milk supply is more established, you can pump or nurse less often. Hand expressing on top of nursing or pumping is a great way to encourage supply in the early days.

If you are mostly pumping, it can be tempting to pump less often when you notice that you get more pumped milk out if you wait more hours, but this can backfire and cause supply to go down. It can also be very tempting to go several very long stretches without milk removal to get rest when combo feeding, because labor and delivery are exhausting on a whole new level. This can also backfire and sabotage lactation.

When you are at capacity, or the most full, you get the most milk that you can make in one sitting. For most people this happens in 4-6 hours. When you allow the breast to fill without frequent draining, you are signaling to your body that you want less milk. With the sensation of fullness there is a hormone produced that signals the body to reduce over-all supply. This hormone is called feedback inhibitor of lactation, or FIL. So, while you would initially see more milk per pump, your daily pump amounts would gradually decline. If you feel very full very frequently the first few days postpartum, your body might start to function such that your baby is not going to need your milk, so it stops making it all-together. Fullness creates a negative feedback loop that dips supply.

Frequency is more important to increasing supply, even when the initial amounts pumped are low. The frequent milk removal signals to the body that you want more milk. Due to the hormonal signaling, frequency and small pump sessions are superior to boosting supply than longer stretches between sessions with initially larger volumes. Frequency creates a positive feedback loop that tells your body to boost supply. It is better to pump 8 times per day for 5 minutes than it would be to pump once per day for 40 minutes. This frequency more closely mimics baby's natural feeding, as newborns tend to eat frequently and in an erratic pattern, or cluster-feed.

The reduction of baby's cluster feeding patterns coincides with our milk regulation hormonal patterns, first around 6 weeks and then again around 12 weeks. The erratic nursing pattern, or lack of a real pattern, is how the baby works with your body in tandem to continue to boost the supply the first 6-12 weeks. The cluster feeding and the sporadic nursing keep the breasts at a low volume compared to capacity, and this is what signals to the body to keep increasing the supply. This is why most lactation professionals discourage parents from putting a breastfed baby on a schedule. This is logistically challenging, as it makes planning around nursing tricky when there is lack of a schedule. As their schedule regulates or becomes more predictable so does the milk because your body starts to get the signal that the baby is more content. If they never seem satisfied the first 4 to 6 weeks, it is because it is their job to act that way. This is part of the design of boosting the supply. You don't start out with a full supply—it is slowly built up over the first few weeks. Even bottle-fed and formula fed babies will try to follow these instincts and cluster feed frequently. Their behavior, as such, is not the best or only indicator of adequate milk supply or transfer. The best indicators are well drained mammae, and baby's adequate diaper output and weight gain.

Even if it seems they are never satisfied, it is important to note that at times they actually are. To know if a baby is sometimes content, you will see their body give you clues. If they are truly never content, this might be a red flag and cause for concern. A content baby usually has open and relaxed hands, gets sleepy and drowsy at the breast after 10-15 minutes or more of nursing, their sucking starts to slow down, and they have good diaper output and weight gain. If they are nursing 30-45 minutes and coming off crying and upset, they may not be getting enough.

A common problem I see in the first few weeks postpartum with efficient milk removal is a simple issue of not offering both breasts every feeding. Many in-patient perinatal healthcare staff will erroneously advise, or parents assume, one breast per feeding is adequate. When milk volume is still low, a baby will generally get more volume if they take both breasts, and the mammae will be more adequately stimulated, thus it is more protective and proliferative to milk supply.

As both breasts start to fill with mature milk, when you offer the first breast and it is its most full, then the initial 2-3 letdowns every 2-3 minutes are a fast flow and the baby gets most of the volume in the first 5-6 minutes. Think of "let-downs" like gushes of flow in the over-all milk flow. They will keep nursing past that initial first few let-downs in order to get more milk and to seek comfort. While on the first breast the baby often dozes off as the rate of flow slows down. This does not mean they are done, or full. The baby will likely have gotten to the fatty hindmilk and drained the breast well if they are starting to doze off. This is when you should at least offer the second side. When you offer the second full breast, they get the faster flowing milk again, and are happy to drink more. The faster flow perks them up, and they get another large volume in the first 5-6 minutes on the second breast. This is how a baby gets more volume spending 10-15 minutes on each breast, rather than 20-30 minutes on one breast. The timing for you and your baby may be shorter, or longer, so these are just general and average guidelines to work with. This habit of offering both sides is not only beneficial to supply regulation but also reduces engorgement discomfort, risk of clogs and mastitis, as well as baby's risks of jaundice, too much weight loss, inadequate gain, and poor blood sugar stabilization.

Once a healthy supply is established, and when a lactating person has a more abundant supply then the baby might stop taking both sides at some of the feeds, or at all of them. It is helpful to always offer both, but do not expect them to always take both. There is usually no reason to worry if they do not always take both sides, but in the early days postpartum you should be consistently offering both sides so that the option is available.

Of course, with variation in personal capacity, you may find over time that because you can hold large volumes of milk at once then you are able to offer one breast per feed and it be adequate. Capacity is how much the breast can hold when full. Doing one breast per feed will take time to build up to, as well as some trial and error to figure out if it is personally feasible for you. Even if your supply can handle it, it may lead to clogs or mastitis. Once supply is more established and capacity determined, you might find that your baby needs only one breast because each of your breasts can hold a full 3-5 ounce feed (or more). You would in that case want them to finish the feed on one side to ensure they got to the fatty hind milk. This can be confusing or hard to guess if your baby needs one or both sides, so do not be afraid to go check in with a consultant to clarify what would be best for you and your baby. Capacity can range from less than an ounce to 20 ounces in each breast so do not feel bad that it takes some educated guessing to figure yours out—that is a huge variety! Throw in variations in refill rate, variation in milk-flow, and variation of the efficiency of your baby nursing--and it can get quite confusing. For example, a very efficient nursling can drain the breasts very quickly, and might get to fatty hind milk in 3-5 minutes. There is no good blanket advice that will work for everyone, such as "10-15 minutes on each breast," because there is so much variation on multiple factors here.

Another important consideration with laying a good foundation is avoiding too much supplementing when combo-feeding. Parents often will sabotage their own lactation relationship early on by frequently topping off a baby with large volumes of pumped milk or formula. This is different from later knowing an appropriate and limited amounts to top off each time due to low supply—it would first need to be established that there is a need and then amounts worked out based on supply estimates from weighed feeds. You would also need to be pumping or hand expressing to off-set the missed stimulation at the breast (if your goal is a full supply). If your goal is combo-feeding with a partial supply and formula, then you still need to be careful and limit top-offs to avoid signaling too much to the body that your milk isn't needed. It can be a bit of a dance to figure out, and hopefully after reading this book you can do so successfully. If not, that is what IBCLC consults are for. You can find a combo-feeding friendly IBCLC to help guide you. You can consider waiting to combo-feed until nursing is sorted out, or it is established that you have a low supply—but it is not entirely necessary.

Parents often fall into a top-up trap when the baby is rooting frequently or seems unsatisfied after eating. Frequent rooting and seeming to not be satisfied after some feeds are innate and instinctive behaviors that serve several biological purposes. A baby might have dozed off but not actually been done suckling. It is unrelated to how nourished or hydrated the baby is, unless you have verified that the baby is not gaining weight well or they have signs of dehydration then you can usually attribute it to normal behavior. Babies are designed to cluster feed and act unsatisfied in order to call your body to boost supply the first 4 to 6 weeks of life. They should be feeding very frequently, and often back to back feeds.

Frequent nursing also forces you to sit still and rest at a time that you need to be; when you are recovering from pregnancy and delivery. They also nurse frequently when they have growth spurts. When you interrupt this pattern with top-off bottles you miss critical signaling to the body to keep boosting supply. Frequent feeding also serves to help keep babies safe, alive, and well cared for when they regularly wake and request your attention.

If you want to know that your baby is getting enough milk then you need to monitor the diaper count daily and the weight gain every few days in the first two weeks, and then weekly in the first 6 weeks. Diaper output should be 1 stool minimum each day (but often more), and 1 wet diaper per day of age up until day 6 when it just generally becomes six or more per day. This means one day 1 we want 1+ wet and 1+ stool, day 2 we want 2+ wet and 1+ stool, day 3 we want 3+ wet and 1+ stool, and so on and so forth. Of note, baby stool is loose and wet, not like adult stools that are firmer and formed.

Weight gain first begins with loss, most babies lose 5-10% of their birth weight (and even more if IV fluids were given during labor). Re-gaining should begin within the first 3-5 days, and be about 0.75 to 2 ounces per day for the first 3-4 months of life. While more than that is okay, less than that can be dangerous to growth and development.

Low Supply

When one does everything to their best ability to lay a good supply foundation and yet they still come up short on volume this is "low supply." This can also happen when laying a good foundation is interrupted by emergencies or sabotaged by bad advice. This would be the camp of people that need to combo-feed by necessity, and not so much by choice. If you find yourself in this situation, it is usually a little more emotionally tumultuous, because it feels like the "choice" behind combo feeding or exclusively breastfeeding was taken away. If this is you, I want to invite you to take time to grieve that. Your lactation grief matters, and I know you are here for so much more than just the "how to" of combo-feeding. The task of laying a good foundation is critical, low supply or not, and once we do that we then have flexibility in our combo-feeding journey. I hope this book empowers you to go forward in this process with knowledge and tools that make the grief a little easier to carry.

Low supply by definition means supply output of the lactating parent does not match a baby's needed milk intake. For example, a parent may make 20-24 ounces per day but have a baby that needs 26-30 ounces per day to thrive. A baby that is thriving is gaining weight appropriately, having plenty of soiled diapers, meeting other growth parameters, and meeting developmental milestones. Having a low supply can change with each child, because of production changes in the lactating parent and different needs for each individual child. For example, a different baby that the same lactating person above feeds later in their life after a subsequent pregnancy might be more petite and thrive with just 22-24 ounces per day, so that person would have a full supply for that baby. The combination of making more milk with each baby and then having a baby with lower metabolic requirements set them up for full supply the second time around. The determination of low supply can be different with each lactation relationship, and even change throughout a relationship. If someone has borderline low supply, they may find that they make enough once their baby starts solids. Also consider, when a baby nurses after 1 year of age they need significantly less milk--so a parent that had low supply the first year may have enough to still go on to nurse past that first year and into toddlerhood. If the nursing relationship is built on soothing, bonding, and connection—the amount of milk is not that important. Nursing can go on for years, even with very minimal supply. The main challenge is establishing and maintaining lactation the first year of life to be able to continue the nursing relationship thereafter.

A true medical low supply is differentiated from a perceived low supply because of the needs of the baby. A person may wish that they made 6 ounces per session so that they had extra to store in the freezer, but they make 4 ounces and none to spare, yet their baby still gains and grows well. They might believe they need 5 or more ounces each pump session, because they are comparing themselves to others online or in mommy groups. This person would have a perceived and not actual low supply. Now, perceived low supply is still stressful! However, we make it a point to differentiate the two only because we find knowledge empowering. We want those that know they have a choice of flexibility to be sure of it, and not be second guessing themselves. We want those with low supply to be validated in their experiences, and to know supplementation is truly needed. There are many examples of perceived low supply, and if your supply is ever in question then you should be seeking an IBCLC.

Now, also consider what a person's capacity is to hold milk in each breast when it is most full. This is surprisingly not directly related to breast size, as most people assume. A breast might be full of mammary tissue and very little fat, having a small appearance. A breast might be full of fat but have very little mammary tissue, having a large appearance. A large breast does not guarantee a large capacity. This is shocking to most large breasted people who struggle with supply. When a large breast does match a large capacity, those people can store much more in one breast than any one baby would ever need at one feeding; I have seen one breast hold up to 20 ounces when full! Alternatively, in any size breast, it is possible that a person may only make 1 ounce in each breast to add up to 2 ounces per feed, and they must feed those 2 ounces every 2 hours to satisfy their baby. This would be 24 ounces per day and likely enough to grow well on for most babies. However, it would require nursing 12 times per 24 hours. A person might consider this a low supply if they are unable to keep up with the demands of this schedule, though technically they might be able to meet their baby's daily nutritional needs. Further still, some people's mammary capacity is even less than an ounce per breast, and yet it is still possible to nurse or pump. There isn't a need to split hairs over it; if you want to supplement regardless of your capacity or supply then we can figure out how!

In general babies eat about 1 ounce per hour, sometimes smaller babies do well with a bit less and sometimes larger babies want a bit more. For a smaller baby 19-24 ounces might be a full supply, and that would be the lower limits of normal. For a larger baby they might want 5 ounce feeds 6 to 7 times per day, so 30-35 ounces would be a full supply for that baby, and that is probably the upper limit of what is typical. Some babies that have higher caloric needs take upwards of 40-50 ounces per day, but this would not be a typical expectation. Bottle fed babies might over-eat a bit, and this often stresses parents out when they think they aren't making enough milk, but actually the baby's caregiver is (accidentally) over-feeding. We will talk more later about a technique called "paced-feeding," that helps prevent that.

Weight gain, overall growth patterns, plenty of soiled diapers, and properly meeting milestones are the important indicators of appropriate intake. Normal intake after 1 month of age can be anywhere from around 2.5 to 5 ounces per feed with breastmilk, and babies eat 8-12 times per day the first few months. The amounts per feed can vary from feed to feed. Sometimes, we just want a snack. Sometimes, we are insatiable and want more than usual. Our babies are the same! Sometimes, babies eat less often, like 5-8 times per day, if they end up taking larger feeds. Sometimes, especially during cluster feeding and growth spurts, babies might eat 16 to 20 times a day. The over-all amount they take most days is pretty stable from ages 1 to 6 months until they start solids. As they start gradually eating more solids this nutritional intake displaces milk intake. Formula amounts are usually slightly higher than breastmilk amounts.

I am going to go slightly off topic here to compare breastmilk to formula, because this sabotages many breastfeeding people when they think they should be producing as much breastmilk as a formula fed baby eats. Formula babies eat larger quantities but less often, due to it digesting more slowly because it is harder to digest. The prevailing theory is that the amount they need continues to increase because it is not a living substance that changes, like breastmilk. When babies get breast milk their intake is more constant, as their gut matures, they hold on to more of the milk. As the months go by, the proteins and other nutrition in the breastmilk also change to better suit the baby's needs. A formula fed or donor milk fed baby might be taking 6-8 ounces per feed between 6-12 months, but a directly breastmilk fed baby would generally not do this. Occasionally, I see babies that want maybe 6 ounces per feed of breastmilk and do well with that, but most will stay in the 2.5 to 5-ounce range. Breastmilk can also be creamier (or have higher fat content) in the same volumes compared to formula. So, if you are offering both breastmilk and formula, don't be surprised if your child wants larger formula bottles versus their breastmilk bottles.

Returning to our topic of low supply, some good news is that most females grow more mammary tissue with each pregnancy. This means a person will most likely increase capacity with each pregnancy, and thus will likely make more milk. However, if you have what is called insufficient glandular tissue, also called IGT for short, you will not likely increase mammary tissue drastically enough with each pregnancy in order to have a full supply. This is because the glandular tissue did not develop enough in puberty, so the proper foundation of cells is not there.

There is also the chance that you have a great capacity but have some hormonal dysregulation, so your breasts are slow to refill with milk. Slow refill means the overall amount for a 24-hour period is insufficient, which can happen despite a normal capacity. An example might be pumping 3 ounces every 4 hours, which is only 18 ounces per 24 hours. The refill being slow would be indicated by still only getting 18 ounces daily even if you pump every 2 hours, getting 1.5 ounces per pump. The breast may have the capacity for 3 ounces, which can be a full feed for some babies, but if you are unable to get the 3 ounces often enough to get a daily total that is sufficient, then it is a slow refill. The refill adequacy is determined by the total of ounces per 24 hours, despite the number of pump or nursing sessions changing.

While my examples are beautiful and simple math, most breasts do not work this way. The circadian rhythm of prolactin is such that it boosts from 12 to 5 AM and bottoms out in the early evening, and thus the milk supply is higher from midnight to noon than it is from noon to midnight. So, the breasts might make 4 to 5 ounces in the nighttime and early morning feeds but make only 2 to 3 ounces in the early evening feeds. The daily total is still the important number to look at.

Too many parents are given the expectation that they will have no problem with supply as long as they work hard enough and make the right choices. Saying a parent is not working hard enough is a cruel and simplified way to lay all blame at their feet when it is likely they have never worked harder at anything in their life, and they are up against many things that they have no control over. We are bombarded from the time we are in-utero until our death with toxins and endocrine disrupters through our diet, lifestyle, and environment. Sometimes the influence of those makes it such that the breast never developed properly to begin with which in turn causes low capacity, or they leave the pituitary or thyroid below optimal functioning which in turn effects milk refill rates. Even those who follow the right protocols and have a knowledgeable and wise support team sometimes still cannot make a full supply due to assaults on their body from many years ago. People with chronic low supply are often not given the thorough medical support they need, even when there is a fixable problem, because there are simply not enough providers trained in lactation medicine. When they need a higher level of care, it is not available.

If you find yourself facing low supply, only you will be able to answer how much effort and how much milk is worth it to you. Sometimes a low supply is a micro supply, totaling only milliliters per day--not in the realm of ounces per day. Any amount of breastmilk provides all the benefits to both the lactating parent and the baby, and nursing is not an all-or-nothing game. No one on your team or in your family can make the call to quit or should suggest you quit. The power of that decision lay entirely within you. Only you know what you can handle or what you personally find worth it.

I find for most people it is reasonable to attempt to maximize their supply based on hormonal norms. For example, trying to bring in any milk after 2 to 3 weeks might be in vain, if your milk never increases beyond a few milliliters. After 2 to 3 weeks, we are no longer hormonally primed to increase mature milk in significant amounts. If frequent pumping or nursing for several weeks did not induce the milk to "come in", then it is not going to. If you are able to get increasing amounts of milk the first 2 to 3 weeks, no matter how slow the increase, then you should be encouraged to keep trying. We are hormonally primed to keep boosting supply for the first 4 to 6 weeks after delivery. Some people are even able to boost supply beyond this. You can take many steps for the first 4 to 6 weeks to keep maximizing supply, and then settle into an easier long-term routine that helps protect the supply, and the nursing relationship if you are feeding directly at the breast. You might also consider doing this up to 12 weeks, or until you no longer see "gains" in your amounts yielded. This might look like doing a breast, bottle, pump plan for the first month, and then cutting out pumping and switching over to just nursing and bottle feeding, or switching to just nursing with an at breast supplementer. A breast, bottle, pump plan means you do all three of those activities at each feeding session for most, if not all, sessions. This routine is usually called "triple-feeding." This is a laborious and exhausting routine, and it is not meant to be done long term.

Some things to consider when contemplating how much breast milk matters to you are the content of the milk, the benefits for the female, and the benefits for the infant. As far as the content, there are millions of antibodies and other important substances in just 1 teaspoon of breastmilk that are not found in formula, so a full supply is not needed to confer the immunological and nutritional benefits. Also, babies are often happy to continue to nurse even with low supply when it is offered with or after some supplemental milk. They can have your milk for dessert instead of the main course, and you can both still get all the benefits of nursing. The benefits of nursing and lactation for a female and baby are largely determined by the length of time you nurse, lactate, or give breastmilk. The benefits are not "dose dependent," meaning a small amount can still provide all the benefits. It matters more that you nurse or provide breastmilk for a set amount of time, versus a set amount of ounces.

Supply regulation, for millions of lactating people, is an ongoing struggle. It is not as rare as most people in the lactation community and the healthcare community assume. While less common than the billions of people with sufficient supply, there are still millions of people experiencing low supply. If the statistics are correct at a conservative estimation, which is arguable, then there are constantly millions of people struggling with milk supply at any given time. Just because this is a low number by comparison, that does not make it a rare occurrence. As rates of hormonal dysregulation exposures rise in our modern society so do the rates of low supply.

It is unfair to put the entire burden of supply regulation on parents, knowing what we know about how common risk factors are, and how little support they receive versus how much they need. The current healthcare system, unfortunately, does put most of the burden on the parents to troubleshoot their own possible contributing factors to their chronic low supply. Support truly needs to be environmental, emotional, economical, logistical, cultural, and personal. We have a long way to go.

If you feel forced into combo-feeding because of low supply, I invite you, again, to process your breastfeeding or lactation grief. That would be sitting with and maybe also exploring in therapy the sadness and grief associated with your lactation journey not being how you imagined it would be. It is a very normal response to grieve what you wanted when it doesn't come to fruition. Connecting with other low supply moms in support groups (online and in person) is a great way to connect, feel validated, and express your grief. Know that you are seen, and your experience is valid.

I explore more extensively in "Can I talk you out of breastfeeding?" background medical information on low supply and why low supply is important (among other challenges of lactation). Please order a copy if you want a more in depth exploration, as it is beyond the scope

of the intention of this particular book.

Supplementation

Supplementation and combo-feeding are closely related concepts but can represent different circumstances. Because they are so closely related people often use the terms interchangeably. Supplementation is most often defined as offering alternative milk sources, like formula and donor milk. Supplementation is often given when a mother has low supply or is working on building up her supply. By the nature of the task, you are combo-feeding if you are supplementing. Some people also use the term to refer to supplementing the act of nursing, regardless of the source of the milk. For example, one might say they are supplementing the baby with hand-expressed milk from its mother.

Combo-feeding is defined in this book as utilizing multiple methods to get milk into a baby, regardless of the source of the milk. This means using multiple tools, but not necessarily multiple sources of milk. For example, a combo-feeding parent might nurse most feeds but then combine that with bottles of their own pumped milk a few times a day, and thus be considered a combo-feeder. They are doing more than just directly nursing from the breast. They are using a combination of tools to feed their baby.

For even those that have a goal of exclusively providing their own breast milk without supplementation of an alternative milk source, some temporary and transitional conditions require that baby be supplemented. Temporary need for supplementation leads into long-term combo-feeding for many parents. Supplementation during the first weeks can serve to supplement what a lactating parent is making, as the name implies. It's purposes may be so that infants do not lose too much weight, do not become dehydrated, do not become too jaundiced, have poor weight gain, or have too low of blood sugars. When a parent uses their own pumped milk to supplement nursing for these reasons, this is when combo-feeding and supplementation can be used interchangeably. However, most people think of formula when they think of the term supplementing.

When assuming that supplementation means it is not the lactating parent's milk then, ideally, the lactating parent is working on boosting their supply if it is within the first 6 weeks postpartum. If you do not pump or hand express during this time frame, while giving supplementation, then you are missing critical stimulation. Your deep inner brain must be stimulated via suckling frequently at the breast to know biologically that an infant has survived labor and delivery, and thus needs feeding. Suckling stimulates the pituitary gland in your brain to make prolactin. Prolactin receptors are laid in the breast in response to the suckling and the high prolactin, and over time this leads the breast to make more milk. This process the first few weeks postpartum is what builds your supply. If you miss laying prolactin receptors while your body is capable immediately postpartum then you risk a chronic low supply. As mentioned in the low supply chapter, you can still meet these requirements and end up with a chronic low supply for other more complex and varied reasons. This is why I promote laying a good foundation, even if your goal is to supplement long-term. It is better to error on the side of caution until you know how robust of a supply you are capable of producing.

The pump or hand expressing will act in place of the suckling babe in the event of supplementation, as every supplement feed offered is a missed opportunity for breast stimulation. If you desire to breastfeed and need to supplement, then in order to not risk your long-term supply you must stimulate the breast every time supplementation is offered. You can achieve both supplementation and breast stimulation simultaneously with at breast supplementers, which we will discuss more in depth later.

Even if you are not aiming for full supply, you still must pump or hand express regularly to get adequate stimulation to keep lactation going. What is defined as "regularly" can vary somewhat due to differences in capacity and refill rate. One person might be able to stimulate every 4-6 hours and succeed at their goals, another may require every 2-3 hours to succeed. Longer stretches come with risks to supply, as well as risks of clogs or mastitis. Figuring out your personal needs will take some experimentation. Around every 4-6 hours should be an absolute maximum between sessions, but every 2-3 hours is more ideal for most. The stimulation between 12 am and 5 am is critical, and you should have at least 1 session during this time frame and it should not be skipped. I will go more in depth on these principles in the "protecting lactation" chapter.

What needs to be more normalized is the expectation of supplementing your baby the first weeks of life, especially for first time parents. To pretend it is unlikely sets us up for emotional turmoil when faced with it in an emotionally heightened and vulnerable time, immediately postpartum. Lactivist campaigns against formula have made many first time parents feel ambivalent about offering it to their babies. However, for tens of thousands of years, we have relied on other lactating people and other animals to help us provide milk for our babies until our mature milk came in. Our species is resilient in being able to share other mammals' milks, and it should be seen as a strength. With modern environmental disruptions it is estimated almost half of modern females having their first child experience their milk coming in later than the 3-5 days most of us are taught to expect. The disruptions might be long term endocrine disruptors like diabetes or short-term delivery disruptions like intravenous fluids. Additionally, infants may not feed very well the first few days or even the first few weeks. For example, if they have birth trauma effecting the mechanics of their latch or jaundice that is making them sleepy. Most families benefit from a temporary and professionally guided supplementation plan because it relieves stress and pressure around caring for the infant and helps ensure the infant is healthy and stable. Studies have reflected that carefully monitored minimal supplementation during the first week can actually lead to better long-term success with establishing and maintaining breastfeeding. This is likely because it helps get babies off to a good physical start and it helps parents have reduced stress around the process.

If you appreciate anticipatory guidance and want more in depth information on all the potential disruptions to lactation and breastfeeding relationships, I highly encourage you to check out my general lactation book "Can I Talk You out of Breastfeeding?" as it goes in depth into all the possible bumps in the road you might face. Its great information, but outside the scope of the intention of this particular book.

The bottom line here is that parents need to know how to supplement in order to succeed with breastfeeding, in the event that it is a needed intervention. Babies need to be well hydrated and have enough nutritional intake to be able to nurse well, so if that is not happening things can go very poorly within just a few days. This is why close follow up is suggested the first week or two postpartum. The key to supply protection is not to supplement without also providing extra stimulation to the breast, which is done with hand expression, pumping, or an at-breast supplementation device. Early supplementation is often a lot more work than long term combo-feeding, but it all gets easier and less demanding as time passes.

Some conditions can sometimes make baby so fragile that they have to temporarily be separated from you to go to the NICU, or in jaundice cases be inside a special blanket with lights or a special bed with lights. You might get a lot of push-back from nurses and doctors who are accustomed to freely giving formula without a second thought when you approach options other than formula to address these concerns. To them formula is just part of a safe, easy, and effective treatment plan. They come from a logical place of wanting to keep your baby safe through using the formula in a medicinal way. This can clash with a strong emotional desire to only provide breast milk, and potentially sabotage lactation if not managed correctly. Neither party is necessarily wrong in their desires, its just a difference of opinion of what is best.

The World Health Organization and other leading health agencies say that formula is a perfectly acceptable alternative milk source when there is a medical need. Formula is biologically the 3rd best option after a lactating parent's own expressed milk and then pasteurized donor milk 2nd, when comparing ingredients. It is one of the best things to offer a hungry baby. Medical needs for supplementation might include jaundice, low blood sugar, and dehydration. I also often make the case that a parent's emotional regulation or mental health needs can be medical needs for offering an infant formula—as a mentally and emotionally well lactating parent is part of the over-all health of the dyad. If you do not have enough breast milk or donor milk, then formula is the next best and safest option whenever not supplementing is not an option. Realistically, ingredients are not the only thing families consider when sorting through infant feeding options. Depending on your personal definition of "best" for your own preferences and needs than formula might be 1st or 2nd on your list, but regardless of how you sort out the differences—formula is perfectly fine to use and formulated to meet your baby's needs.

While waiting for your milk to come in is not necessarily a medical need for supplementation itself, supplementing can prevent some medical issues from arising during a vulnerable time. Many parents are comfortable with and happy to supplement minimally while waiting for the milk to start to flow in larger volumes because of this. Your healthcare team is watching for signs that the baby might need supplemented, because scary things can happen if we miss the cues. When a baby does not get enough milk their blood sugar can drop, and in extreme cases if it drops low enough it can lead to seizures. The baby may become dehydrated, which if severe enough can be a threat to their life. It may feel sometimes like supplementation is pushed because healthcare providers do not want to risk these awful things happening when it is perfectly safe to supplement and avoid risking them. Other than those physical needs it might also meet the needs of the parents to feel reassured about how well their baby is being fed. It can also take some of the pressure off of the lactating parent. Babies who are well hydrated and have good energy levels after a little bit of supplementation will often do better at the breast. There is research and anecdotal evidence that early and minimal supplementation in conjunction with lactation support actually helps parents meet their long-term breastfeeding goals.

While it is likely true that milk has taken about 3 to 5 days to come in since the beginning of human existence, it is also true that our lifestyles and risk factors for delayed milk are generally vastly different today compared to thousands of years ago. In days passed we used to have several lactating people physically close to us that might help nurse our babies until our mature milk came in, or we would maybe borrow from the family goat. We are a resilient species, and part of the reason for that is our flexibility in our diet. I think we need to keep that in mind when formulating infant feeding plans.

Today, most of us have formula and donor milk, rather than close lactating relatives or family cows. Formula can help keep your baby alive and well, and does not mean that you will not still meet your breastfeeding goals. If the idea of formula is being brought up and you are planning to breastfeed exclusively then a lactation consultant needs to be on the healthcare team that is making plans and decisions. You will need to follow a plan that you make with the help of a lactation consultant to protect your supply.

If donor milk might be an option for your baby, you will probably want to talk to your partner about it, if you have one. Some people find they prefer formula to donor milk, or vice versa. It is important to sit and think about your feelings around which supplemental milk to use when you are calm and not under pressure to decide. You will also have to decide whether to only use pasteurized donor milk from a milk bank, or if you are going to engage in peer to peer sharing. Peer to peer milk sharing can be friends you know or facilitated through online social media milk sharing groups. Donor milk has risks, just like formula, and usually comes with a different set of emotional responses when you consider giving another person's milk to your baby. There are also financial considerations, if you cannot get pasteurized donor milk covered by your insurance it is very expensive. Peer to peer milk is usually donated in exchange for pumping parts rather than purchased and this is to remove incentive to water it down or add volume by adding alternative milks in order to gain more profit. Some benefits of donor milk include involving other caregivers in feeding, and the baby getting a larger variety of antibodies and stem cells to strengthen his immune system and body, overall.

While using formula is not without risk, I believe the risks are misinterpreted or exaggerated sometimes to meet lactivist agendas. Some studies show that infants who are not breastfed have higher rates of ear infections, stomach bugs, lung disease, obesity, diabetes, cancer, and SIDs. However, take that with a grain a salt because removing confounding variables (or other influencing factors) or looking at relative risk makes those differences negligible. The myth that formula feeding effects IQ, for example—has been debunked. There are some scary truths however, such as that premature infants who do not get any breastmilk have an increased risk of bowel death. Any human milk (via nursing, pumping, or donor) that you can provide reduces all of these risks (regardless of how small they might be), especially in the first 6 months of life.

Not to be forgotten are the risks and benefits to the lactating female body. Females who do not lactate have higher rates of breast, ovarian and colorectal cancer, obesity, diabetes, hypertension, osteoporosis, and metabolic syndrome. The longer you lactate, the more protection your body derives from these ailments. The benefits are not dependent on the amount of milk made, but rather the length of time that milk is made.

From the data we have I think we can reasonably draw some logical conclusions. It is my belief that any lactation relationship is providing all the protection and all the benefits to both the lactating parent and the baby, and we should be more flexible in allowing formula to help us meet the demands of infant feeding. When we leave it out as an option then we miss the gifts it is offering.

Keep in mind that not considering the need to supplement can make it feel like a much heavier decision when you are freshly postpartum and more sensitive than usual. You might have an idea to start combo-feeding a month or two into nursing, but the reality might be that you need to start right away. In this case it is wise to hope for the best outcome but prepare for alternatives. It can negatively influence when you later reflect on the first few days of your baby's life if you feel pushed or rushed into the decision. Once you decide to supplement, or accept that you might need to, you will also have to consider the tools you will use to supplement with. The next chapter explores different feeding tools.

Device Options

Choices for supplementation include spoons, bottles, syringes, cups, at breast supplemental nursing systems, finger feeding, and tube feeding. When the need to supplement is in the first few days and in smaller quantities it can make sense to use the smaller tools versus the bottles but it is okay to start with and only use bottles, if that is your preference.

Spoons are excellent for collecting colostrum via hand-expression and then tipping directly into baby's mouth—especially the first few days. Small syringes with curved tips are great for the first few days too, because you can have the baby suckle the breast or a finger while syringing some supplement into their cheeks. Finger feeding can be done with a syringe and tube set-up as well. Very small cups are also used worldwide to help pour small amounts into baby's mouth to get them to drink. This can be especially helpful if you have a baby with oral aversions who is resistant to latching onto anything.

Supplemental nursing systems at the breast were invented to help adoptive mothers stimulate milk supply but can also be helpful for parents with low supply, premature infants, or babies who are full term but small for their gestational age. They enable you to bring the baby to the breast while getting a supplement at the same time. They are made up of a reservoir and tube. The reservoir might be a bottle, bag, or syringe that then connects to a tube. The reservoir holds the supplement and the tube tucks into the baby's mouth once they are suckling on the breast. This encourages the baby to keep suckling on the breast because they get an increased flow from the supplement. The supplemental nursing system is often reserved by professionals as an option for those we know will be supplementing for several months and whose parents prefer to keep the baby at breast rather than using a bottle. An at breast system is not a great option for a baby that cannot transfer milk effectively, as that would risk not getting adequate breast stimulation to protect lactation. Additionally, some parents find they prefer to use bottles because of the difficulty keeping the tubing in baby's mouth once they are more active. If a parent has a micro-supply or very slow flow, but they want to keep the baby at breast then they would be a great candidate for incorporating the at breast supplementing systems. A parent in these circumstances might do bottles part time and at breast supplementers part time.

Of course, it is possible to use a variety of different combo-feeding tools simultaneously, depending on your preferences and needs. Circumstances may dictate different caregivers use different tools. In the first few weeks most babies are flexible on what supplemental device they will accept. Sometimes, babies only accept certain tools from certain caregivers. For example, some babies only take bottles from their father, but will not take one from their mother. Keep all of the options in mind if you need to combo-feed as what you prefer, and what your baby might accept, may change over time.

Once you are giving more than an ounce at a time to supplement, typically after the first few days, then some of these options can be cumbersome and not worth the minimal risk of nipple or flow preference that is present when you supplement with bottles. Many babies are happy to continue nursing even when they also need to supplement part time, regardless of the method, as nursing is an instinctive and desired behavior for human infants.

Many families find they prefer to keep some bottle feeding in their routine once they have experienced the benefits of combo feeding. It allows more partner involvement, more rest for the breastfeeding parent, more flexibility for the whole family, and reduced stress around achieving and maintaining a full supply. When choosing a bottle there are so many options out there, it can get quite confusing. If you introduce bottles early enough there should not be too much issue with bottle refusal. The ideal time to introduce it is within the first few weeks of life, when suckling drive is high.

It is important to choose a bottle that functions like a breast when inside the baby's mouth, rather than looks like a breast when outside of the baby's mouth. For example, the soft silicone of a bottle nipple does not respond enough to the pressure and shape of a baby's oral cavity for the breast shaped bottle nipples to be a good fit. A breast shaped bottle nipple outside of the mouth does not behave like an actual nipple and breast tissue when inside the mouth. The shape and texture of breast-shaped bottle nipples often discourage a good over-all latch and keeps the baby's mouth very shallow on the nipple. The nipple should have a gradual slope and be soft and flexible, to allow for a deep latch. A deep latch is critical to nursing success, and should be encouraged with the bottle rather than the bottle creating bad habits. The sides of a bottle nipple should look more like a curved banana versus the arches of a rainbow. I will expand more on bottle choice and use in the next topic, covering "paced-feeding."

Paced Feeding

Paced feeding is a popular phrase amongst lactation professionals, and with good reason. Bottle feeding is the most commonly used tool for combo-feeding parents. It is convenient and just makes sense for most families. Using this batch of paced-feeding suggestions, you can (most of the time) avoid a bottle preference.

Often, a baby with difficulty getting milk flow at the breast will develop a preference for bottles--if given the option. This is often mistakenly called nipple confusion. Babies are not confused—they want the milk the easiest and most comfortable way they can get it. What they develop would be more aptly named a flow preference. When they have an easier time getting a flow and getting full from the bottle, they will prefer it. Preferring the easiest way to get food is likely a survival instinct. Using a slow flowing bottle nipple and paced feeding techniques can somewhat help a baby to not prefer the bottle over the breast.

A baby that can latch comfortably and can stimulate fast gushes of milk via the let-down is going to be happy at the breast. A baby will also be happy at the breast if milk flow is abundant, even without much effort on their part to draw the milk out. If a baby is either sleeping at the breast after a short period of suckling or angry at the breast, then they are signaling that there is a problem with flow. Many parents think they exhibit these behaviors because they are waiting for or demanding a bottle. These issues could arise because a baby cannot efficiently remove the milk, or it may be because the milk flow is too slow or low to keep them happy and interested--or it could be both.

Many parents also mistake normal milk stimulating actions as refusal of the breast, and rush too quickly to give the bottle. All mammals pop on and off the nipple, shake their head, and fuss and "paw" at the breast or teat. It looks like the baby is pushing the breast away, but they are trying to knead it. Shaking their head is not saying "no" it is how they help stimulate the nipple to an erect position. This is all on purpose and helps stimulate the letdown. As long as baby is not angry it is important to let them exhibit this natural and instinctive behavior on the breast. I would highly encourage you to watch videos online of baby-led latching, as well as puppies and kitties nursing, to get an idea of what I mean.

Bottle preference developing when the nursing parent is at work for many hours a week is usually due to the caretaker making the bottle too fast, too large, and too often. The parent cannot keep up with the overfeeding because it is outside of the biological norm, and baby becomes accustomed to the new changes and prefers them because they are getting full faster and easier. The pace, frequency, and volume being too much are not because the parent is failing to pump enough but because the caretaker is offering a large bottle with a fast flow every time they fuss. Discussing "paced" feeding techniques and appropriate amounts with your infant's caregiver should take place as early as possible to help manage expectations to avoid unintentional sabotage of the breastfeeding relationship. This is an important discussion to have, sometimes repeatedly, with whomever will be feeding your baby when you are at work. They will need to know what resources they have, tools they can use, and skills they need to develop to soothe a fussy baby, other than just giving them a bottle. They will also need to know how to pace-feed a bottle, when they do offer it.

Another helpful tip for mimicking the breast on the bottle is using more narrow and gradual sloped nipples. Think more of the shape of a cup versus a bowl. Think of how the nipple is inside the mouth versus what it looks like before the baby latches to it. The wide breast shaped nipples keep babies from being able to latch deeply. The narrow-sloped nipples allow baby to latch deeply, like they do to the breast.

Pacing a feeding means you are trying to match not only the pace but also the sensations of nursing. The nipple level choice should be a very low one, such as preemie or newborn. To continue this, nipples need replaced every 2-3 months, as they wear out. The amount in the bottles should be consistent with what a baby would typically nurse from the chest, so 2.5-5 ounces for most people. If they still want to suckle, due to a high suckling drive, then offer a pacifier for about 5-10 minutes to allow the milk to settle. It takes about 10 minutes for the brain to realize the stomach is full, and babies often just like to keep suckling for comfort. If they still show hunger signals after that, then very slowly and gradually try larger bottles, about 0.5 ounce bigger for 2-3 days. Try to match the bottle to what you pump, and give the baby more frequent bottles, versus giving the baby large bottles less frequently. Try not to give baby big bottles that don't match pumped output closely. If your pump output is much greater than what the baby will take, you might see an IBCLC to do a weighed feeding or two, and estimate what baby typically draws from the breast. This might look like giving 3 ounces every 2 hours versus 6 ounces every 4 hours. A baby should take about 1-1.5 ounces per hour on average, and you slowly build up to this rate the first 2-4 weeks and then it should stay pretty stable from 1 to 6 months when solids are introduced.

The baby is positioned almost upright, and the bottle is held almost horizontally, meaning level with the ground. The baby's head and bottle make a very shallow "V" shape. This would be compared to holding the baby laid back, and the bottle almost vertically, or upright, creating a "T' shape. The baby should be burped frequently, every 1-2 ounces consumed. The arm you hold the baby in while feeding should also be switched sides halfway through, much like they switch sides when nursing. This helps with pacing the feed, and their visual development. The feed should take about as long as an average nursing session. This helps the baby not get used to getting too full too fast. It helps prevent over-feeding and helps avoid bottle preference. The frequency of feeding should match the frequency of nursing sessions, so every 2-3 hours for most babies (or even more often if cluster feeding).

There are many helpful youtube videos and images online if you need visual aid for understanding this concept, or to show other caretakers in your baby's life that will be helping bottle feed. It is important that they know that what is natural and normal is for babies to want smaller more frequent feeds, and that wanting this does not equate a need to keep increasing bottle amounts. Having an overly full tummy regularly will dysregulate a baby's natural ability to self-regulate their food and liquid intake. It is good for their bodies to be able to eat when hungry and stop when full, and not be over-fed in an attempt to get them to eat less often.

Formula

When working out which formula to use from the start, you first need a bit of education on it. Sometimes the formula you end up using has more to do with your child's preference than anything else. Going into the decision-making process armed with some knowledge will take some of the guess-work and stress of it away. Rest assured, formula has had a lot of time and love poured into it's science over the years so that your baby can thrive on it.

Formula has the same main macro and micro ingredients as breastmilk. Those macros being carbohydrates or sugars (mainly lactose), proteins (whey and casein), and fats. Micros being vitamins and minerals, and sometimes some extras like probiotics. Vitamins and minerals will be generally the same in different formulas, so that they meet infants' needs. The "extras" are added ingredients that often make formula more expensive and they aim to make the formula more like breastmilk, so they are probably not even necessary if you are combo-feeding with your own milk or donor milk--because you are already providing the extra benefits of breastmilk that the added formula extras are trying to mimic. Some things will probably never be replicated in formula like stem cells, hormones, antibodies, flavors from the lactating parent's diet, and other bio-active components. Yet, some formulas have more of some of the micro-ingredients than breastmilk does, such as vitamin D and iron. So, combo fed babies don't need supplements for those things, where exclusively breastmilk fed infants do. Combo-feeding can really be the best of both worlds.

You might have been surprised to see most formulas contain a main ingredient of lactose as its carbohydrate source. Common myth among parents (and even professionals) is that often babies are lactose intolerant, and this is used to explain difficulty with breastmilk or formula. It is really a convenient myth that is used to avoid the hard work of investigation when feeding is going poorly. Lactose intolerance would have to be a very rare issue in human babies, as it is the main sugar found in breastmilk. Lactose is something most children grow out of being able to digest around the time they lose their milk-teeth (or baby teeth), but as infants we are perfectly suited as we make a special enzyme called "lactase" that breaks down lactose. Lactase is also found in human milk, to help the infant digest the lactose. Lactose intolerance in infants is very rare, otherwise we would not have lasted long as a species.

Lactose is made up of smaller parts called glucose and galactose. Lactose intolerance is the absence of enough of the enzyme lactase to break down the lactose into its smaller parts. Most adults are lactose intolerant, as we generally stop producing lactase as we age and especially if we stop ingesting dairy products. Galactosemia is a rare condition where babies are born without the ability to convert the galactose to anything else and it builds up in the body and causes severe problems. Lactose free formula or lactose reduced formulas might be prescribed to your baby if they have either of these conditions. Other sugar or carbohydrate sources are used for these formulas. Reduced lactose formulas often have corn syrup, and this can cause looser stools. Corn syrup therefore helps with constipation, but if this is an issue you should actually look to the proteins first. If a baby has trouble with constipation from proteins, switching to a different sugar might just mask the problem by getting rid of the constipation. They would likely still have other signs of poor digestion, however.

Carbohydrates are a main source of energy in breastmilk, so formula is made to mimic that. Sources of carbohydrates vary, but you can find formulas that use lactose, which is the main carb in breastmilk. Other sources might be maltodextrin, sucrose, corn syrup, or brown rice syrup.

While most animal milk uses lactose for its main sugar, types of proteins and amounts of fat ratios are what is so different about different mammal's milks. Mammals are animals that have mammary glands and make milk, so that includes humans. Humans are what are called "carry mammals" that are born immature and need to be fed very frequently, our milk has relatively low fat and protein compared to other mammal types. We are grouped with monkeys and kangaroos on this (amongst others). Then, there are "follow mammals" that their babies are born a bit more mature and they can stand and walk right away so they follow their mamas and feed frequently; their milk is also lower in fat and protein compared to other mammals but not as low as carry mammals. Examples of these babies are cows, giraffes, horses, and elephants. Carry and follow mammals feed frequently all day and all night, and they are not separated from their mammas for the first few months of life (or longer). The other two mammal groups are "cache" and "nest," they have higher fats and proteins and can leave their babies for longer periods in nests and safe spaces like caves or burrows, while they go off and hunt or gather food. Cache animals have the highest fat and protein in their milk, and the most mature brains; they include deer and rabbits. They can be separated for upwards of 12 hours at a time. Nest animals are next on the maturity rating, and have slightly lower fats and proteins in their milk. They can be separated 4-6 hours at a time. Examples of mammals that are nest animals are cats, dogs, and wolves. Highest to lowest the order is cache, nest, follow, then carry. All this to say, in order for our species to thrive on another species' milk, some tweaking needs to be done. It is not only the fat and protein ratios but specific micro-nutrient ratios that need adjusted in order to be safe for baby humans to flourish on.

So, if we go further into breaking down the differences then we see that the ratios of types of proteins are different for different mammals. Proteins are like a construction crew for the body—they build, transport, and convert substances as needed to keep the body growing and functioning. The two main protein types are whey and casein, the main difference being how quickly they digest. Whey protein is generally easier to digest for carry mammals, which is why it is naturally higher in concentration in mama carry mammal's milks. Protein in carry mammal milk is usually about 80% whey protein and 20% casein at first and it eventually evens out to a 50% each ratio as the baby mammal ages. Protein in follow mammals is about 20% whey and 80% casein. Part of why it seems that formula "sits heavier" or "lasts longer" in baby's bellies is because of the extra steps it takes a human to break down follow mammal milk proteins. This is also why sometimes formula is harder on a baby's gastrointestinal tract, and they get more gastrointestinal symptoms with formula versus breastmilk. Some formulas intentionally add more whey to help with this. You should be able to find a whey and casein ratio on the formula container. Ratios closer to human milk ratios, in theory, are easier for babies to digest.

Breaking things down even further, casein can be type A1 or A2. Human milk contains A2, and follow-mammal milk has both A1 and A2. Goat's make less A1 than cows, which is why some babies seem to do better on goat milk formulas versus cow milk formulas. In sensitive formulas whey proteins might be added, specific sub-types of casein proteins might be removed, or proteins might be broken down. This is all so that they are more easily processed in the infant's gastrointestinal tract. The A2 formulas are a great option for babies who are sensitive, yet not intolerant or allergic to milk-proteins in traditional formulas.

A word you might see on formula containers is "hydrolyzed" and this means "broken down." This can be further divided to partially hydrolyzed or extensively hydrolyzed, and the need for either would be determined by an infant's sensitivity to the proteins. A partially hydrolyzed formula would be good for a sensitivity, while extensively hydrolyzed might be needed for a severe sensitivity or outright allergy.

Protein in all forms can be broken down even further to its most basic form—amino acids. Amino acids are the building blocks of the proteins. There are special hypo-allergenic formulas that break the milk proteins down to this level, or closer to it. They are best suited to babies with severe milk protein allergies and rare medical conditions making digestion of formula dangerous or life-threatening. This is the next step if extensively hydrolyzed formulas are still causing issues, or there are signs of allergic response to the formula. Other hypo-allergenic formulas may use different sources of proteins such as pea and soy. You would only use these types of formulas under direction of your child's healthcare provider. Specialized formulas can be very expensive. Sometimes specialized formulas are prescribed to have insurance off-set the expense, or assistance programs might be available to off-set the cost.

Fats in formula are sourced from added vegetable oils as well as the animal fats from the milk itself, when it is a dairy based formula. Fat provides fatty acids. They are building blocks for health and bodily functions, and we can't make our own of some of the fatty acids There are many types of fatty acids in breast milk so formula companies often use a blend of oils to try to mimic the composition. Some oils you might see in formula are sunflower, safflower, soybean, palm, coconut, or rapeseed. Palm oil can be constipating and is not considered an ingredient that is mother-earth friendly. If your baby's only problem with formula is constipation, you might just try eliminating that ingredient.

Additional ingredients added for benefits similar to breastmilk include probiotics, prebiotics, DHA, and sometimes others. As formula science advances, we add these things as we can to make them more comparable. Probiotics and prebiotics are important to all human's gut health. They are essential for digestion and immune system support. DHA is an omega fatty acid that is present in human breastmilk, but not in cow milk. It is really helpful for human brain development!

Living in an international economy, we must also consider popular European formulas. There are also "toddler" formulas to consider. What one must look at with these alternatives is if the regulation process of these formulas is as strict as or stricter than what the FDA requires for infant formulas in the USA. Some of the European or toddler formulas are equivalent in ingredients, and nutrient requirements. It would benefit you to discuss with your child's healthcare provider, your IBCLC, or get some information online for comparisons. I won't address specific brands or formulations here, as that is beyond the scope of intention for this book and by the time you read it, some of them may not even be on the market anymore. My aim here is to give general education on formula as a product available for feeding your baby. Much of the work here has already been done on formula comparisons, and continues to be investigated by professionals; so, you don't need to re-invent the wheel, but do find a reputable source for your information. As such, with so many safer options, I would highly discourage home-made formulas, except in emergency cases where no other food source is available.

Signs your baby might need a special sensitive formula or a change in formula are constipation, excessive fussiness, reflux, excessive gas, discomfort, straining with gas or bowel movements, severe or widespread eczema, poor weight gain, congestion, mucous in the stool, or blood in the stool. Infrequent bowel movements, gas, and minor reflux can be normal findings in babies, so its important to look at the whole picture and see if things are excessive; these three alone are usually not enough for a diagnosis and maybe some other trouble-shooting needs to happen with your IBCLC. In just one example a triad of excessive gas, low supply, and poor weight gain might be a latch and transfer issue caused by oral tethers and not at all a formula issue! When combo-feeding there are so many variables. You need someone to look at all the angles of your feeding relationship to help you troubleshoot. Sometimes you just need someone very familiar with babies to let you know if your baby's level of gas is normal or worrisome. Sometimes, you need help discerning between infrequent stooling versus constipation. Professionals can help you troubleshoot these baby issues and concerns; it's what we live for!

These signs and symptoms in baby might also be signs you need to cut certain foods from your diet. If you are cutting something from the diet you also want to cut it from the formula, like dairy proteins. Formula and food intolerance trouble-shooting is really outside the scope of this books intentions, and should be based on a thorough history, sometimes stool or blood testing, and discussion with a qualified healthcare provider. There's really lots of details about formula that we just don't explore here. I just wanted to give you the basics to get you started in your knowledge of formula, and some red flags to watch out for. If your baby is not tolerating milks (breast or formulas), they need worked up for more serious conditions like MSPI (milk soy protein intolerance), CMPI (cow milk protein intolerance), and FPIES (food protein induced enterocolitis syndrome).

If you do explore switching formulas on your own, know what is normal. When introducing a new formula—give it a few weeks to settle. With a brand new digestive system your baby will have poop changes, changes in their gas, or change their habits around eating (such as how frequently they want to eat). When a baby has a fussy period (as they sometimes do), you don't need to panic and change up your formula. Ride the waves of baby temperaments being up and down. If a negative sign or symptoms sticks around more than a few weeks, consider a formula switch or look to your own diet. If you have clear indication to switch, don't wait it out. This would be if your pediatrician advises you to, there is repeatedly blood in the stool, if your baby has a diagnosed allergy, or if there is a recall. Getting professional help on formula changes can help prevent problems being made worse and help prevent you from spending extra money on more expensive formula types if it isn't needed. Same thing with changing your diet; getting some professional insight might save you from cutting dairy for a year if you don't actually have to!

In the formula section, I also wanted to address a question that comes up frequently for combo feeding families, and that is whether to mix formula with breastmilk or not. For those in the camp that say not to mix, the main concern is wasted breastmilk. If your baby does not finish a formula bottle it has to be tossed within an hour, but breastmilk you can wait a couple of hours (or around the next feed). This is because the living antibodies in breastmilk help keep harmful bacteria counts down, and formula doesn't have this advantage. Therefore, a mixed bottle has potential to end up with waste of breastmilk. Now, if you're pretty confident your baby will drink the whole bottle then mix away! Or if you aren't particularly concerned with waste because you have an abundant supply, then by all means mix it up. If you want to avoid wasting any breastmilk just offer it in a separate bottle (or from the tap) prior to offering the formula. You can also mix your own milk with donor milk, as a study has shown this inoculates the milk and more of what is tailored to your baby's environment in your milk gets replicated in the donor milk as time passes. This is because breast milk is a living and adaptable substance.

A helpful tool for combo feeding is using a large pitcher for collecting and prepping milk. You can combine everything into one pitcher, top it with a pouring spout accessory, and keep it in the fridge. You can collect all your pumped milk in one place—the pitcher. When prepping formula you can prep for 24 hours at a time, mixing it all in one big pitcher. When thawing donor milk, it's also good to feed for 24 hours from thawing, so you can combine it all in one large pitcher. If you want to get even more simplified, put all the milks combined in one pitcher, and pour from it as needed. It's only once the baby's lips touch the nipple that the clock starts for it only being good for an hour (if formula is in the mix). So, in theory just the 2-5 oz at each individual feed is what you have to time for being good for one hour. If you have just donor and pumped milk, its good for 2 hours (so possibly until the next feed). It keeps things simple and streamlined to put everything in one place, and helps out other caregivers. They know just one place to get the milk for the baby from, and they don't mess with the rest of your system and accidentally use the wrong thing out of order or at the wrong time.

Protecting Lactation

Even if you start combo feeding from the beginning, it is still important to follow some guidelines of laying a healthy supply foundation. Supplement should be offered pretty minimally at first, while ensuring that the breast is stimulated via pumping, hand-expressing, or nursing every 2-3 hours (at a minimum), so around 8-12 times a day. There is wiggle room that lies in the fact that you can most likely safely skip a few sessions in one long stretch for 4-6 hours every 24 hours and still protect your supply. Further wiggle room comes in to play if you go into the situation knowing you are comfortable sacrificing full supply for the goal of combo feeding. In this case your minimum beginning pump or nursing sessions might be more like every 3-4 hours. If you have a larger capacity, you might even go for every 4-6 hours, but beware that going too many long stretches might send the signal to the body to dry up. This would be disastrous for someone with low capacity, because they would constantly be making an abundance of the feedback inhibitor of lactation hormones. For this reason, I highly discourage first time parents to risk sacrificing supply until they are aware of their supply limitations in general. If this is not your first time breastfeeding then you have some background data to guide you on what your breasts are capable of. There will be a minimum for your body that you need to maintain in order to not dry up. For each person that can be different, and you will actually need to experiment with it some. I would not recommend expressing milk less than every 2-4 hours at first while you figure things out, to avoid drying up. In addition, I'd highly encourage cluster feeding or power pumping once a day in the first few weeks to protect and continue to boost lactation.

Some main things you are trying to avoid when combo-feeding are offering so much supplement that your baby won't nurse, or not getting adequate breast stimulation to the point that your milk dries up. These are some of the main points of the balancing act with combo-feeding.

You don't have to focus very much on how much milk you make when you are combo feeding, because the goal is just to keep the lactation relationship going. The focus is really more on timing, stimulation, and the nursing relationship than it is about amounts. This can be a huge relief when you have low supply, and also quite the relief for every lactating parent to not be the sole nutrition provider for their baby.

When pumping on top of nursing on demand you might express 15-60 milliliters (or 0.5-2 ounces) at each pump session, or less with a low supply. If exclusively pumping you might express 60 to 150 milliliters (or 2 to 5 ounces) each pump session, or less with a low supply. For conversion, 30 milliliters is equal to about an ounce. Those with over-supply and higher capacity can expect even more. While its helpful to know these amounts, its not really relevant to combo-feeding success, because the goal should be to extend the lactation relationship, not necessarily get the most breastmilk. Though, if your personal goal is to supply as much breastmilk as possible, you need to pay close attention to what is required to build up a milk supply. I personally believe most people who combo feed should not focus on that. Part of the benefit and joy of combo-feeding is not having to focus on the amount of milk you make. It can really set you up for frustration if you start putting amounts on your goals. The body responds with so much variation, pump to pump and day to day, that it can be psychologically difficult if we don't meet those self-imposed goals.

The numbers you do want to focus on are trying to narrow down what your breast capacity might be, or at how many hours between feeding or pumping sessions your capacity is reached. Focusing on capacity is important because of a very important biological feedback loop of hormones that can help or hurt your lactation goals. You will want to focus on those numbers, as well as length of time goals. Setting a 6 week goal can get you through supply initiation and supply building. Setting a 12 week goal can get you through the fourth trimester. Setting a six month goal can really help you push through a four month sleep regression. Goals help you push through inevitable hurdles.

It is very important to protecting lactation long-term that you understand the feedback inhibitor of lactation hormone. As the breasts fill, more and more of the feedback inhibitor of lactation hormone is made. A very full breast many times a day makes a lot of this hormone! It signals to the rest of the lactation production regulators that you over-all are wanting less milk. It is meant to help regulate supply. If we make too much of this too often, we dry up! This is partly what facilitates weaning as our baby nurses less and less often when they take in more and more solids. Having your mammae feel very full very often is a bad thing for trying to protect lactation. It does the opposite—it sabotages it! It is important to pay attention to this when working out your combo feeding routine. Routines are going to be different for each person, as capacity and refill rate varies so vastly.

There are several general ways you can approach protecting lactation when nailing down your combo feeding routine. Approaches to combo feeding can involve the following: using bottle feeds for snacks, focusing supplementing when supply naturally dips every day in the evening, using the at breast supplementer, supplementing at every other feeding, parallel pumping some feeds, offering a bottle before during or after each feed, nursing for comfort only, combining your pumped and supplemented milk in bottles together, and utilizing pumping to get breaks from nursing. You can do one method all day and a less stressful method at night. You can do one method while working, one method while at home, and yet another at night. There is no wrong way, only your way. As long as you stick to moving milk in the mammary glands regularly and at peak prolactin production, from 12 to 5 AM, then you should be able to keep lactation going!

Using supplements as snacks allows the lactating parent to get a break. If your baby is taking 3-5 ounces for feeds, snacks would be 1-2 ounces at a time. This is great for introducing and maintaining bottle skills for parents that want to mostly nurse but are going to be separated from their babies due to work or shared custody arrangements. You can start offering bottle snacks right away! This helps avoid taking too much away from breast stimulation without making things overly complicated. Using a snacking method successfully would require spacing out the snacks throughout the day, and avoiding creeping up in amounts. Letting the baby have small snack bottles can be an option for getting baby some bottle skills, regardless of the long-term routine you settle with.

Supplementing a few times in the evening when supply is naturally lower is a great way to get a big chunk of time where you can take a break from nursing. Combo feeding does not have to be a 50/50 split, it can just be a few supplemental feeds a day. You might only offer bottles from around 5 PM to 10 PM, when prolactin (and thus supply) naturally dips. This would be opposite to the prolactin peak around 12 PM to 5 AM, where milk making is more abundant. Midnight to early morning is the worst time to skip feeds because emptying the mammae during this time frame sets your supply for the next 24-72 hours. Additionally, the increase of milk synthesis makes you more likely to get clogs and mastitis if you skip feeds in this timeframe. Early evening, however, is a prime opportunity to get some rest and take a break from being the feeding caretaker. Your mammary glands are refilling more slowly so you are less likely to face issues with being painfully full and less likely to develop clogged ducts from the milk not being moved frequently enough. You can go 4 to 6 hours without draining the breast easier at this time versus at other times of day, and it should not have an over-all negative effect on your supply.

Another way might be doing every other feeding nursing, and every other feeding a supplement. This would be more of a 50-50 or evenly split arrangement. Babies eat so frequently that you'd likely still be nursing every few hours, and getting enough stimulation to keep lactation going, at least in the first few weeks before feeds start spacing out. This is one plan where full supply is risked. If you lay a good foundation, it might not ultimately be an issue to only be stimulating the breast every 3-4 hours versus every 1.5 to 3 hours, which is what exclusively nursed babies sometimes do. If your baby eats every 3 hours then you risk going 6 hours between breast stimulations and your body may not respond well to that. It really all depends on your baby's appetite and your mammary tissue's storage capacity. Some one with larger storage capacity might be able to stimulate the mammae every 6 hours with a near full supply yet alternatively for some this would cause a huge dip in supply but might still be enough to keep lactation going, still for others it might cause them to completely dry up. Again, when you are combo feeding the amounts of milk aren't really usually the goal we focus on—but rather the goal is length of time that we keep lactation going. That doesn't make amounts totally irrelevant! We need to know our max capacity and max time between breast stimulations to safely keep lactation going. This is not just for supply maintenance but also to avoid clogs and mastitis.

Another approach to combo feeding is using pumping to get a break from nursing, or to exclusively pump. This is especially feasible when you invest in a wearable or mobile pump. It can feel very liberating to just go about your business while someone else sits with the baby and a bottle. It's one reason many exclusive pumpers enjoy pumping and bottle feeding versus at the chest feeding for every session. You can focus extra pump sessions in the morning when milk is more abundant, and use the evening to have a more relaxed schedule.

If you have over-supply and make a full feed amount in each breast, you might pump one side and nurse on the other, and have someone else give that pumped milk at the next feed while you skip the session and catch a nap or run an errand. Nursing one side and pumping the other simultaneously is called "parallel pumping," and while often thought of to utilize to help boost supply, it is also a great method to help set aside milk for later! This particular scenario might look like parallel pumping every 4-6 hours, and yielding about 3-5 ounces (or more) in each breast at each of those sessions. One side goes directly into baby, and the other side's yield is set aside for later. Someone with such a high capacity would have the luxury of pumping or nursing less often without risk of too much Feedback Inhibitor of Lactation hormone sabotaging supply. The baby would then get every other feed at the breast, and every other feed a bottle.

On the opposite side of the spectrum would be with a low supply, offering more supplement than your own milk. If you are needing to give a lot of donor milk or formula, it can come down to needing to do this at every feed. You might offer the bottle first, then let the baby finish the feed at the breast. We might call this "having dessert" at the breast. This would allow frequent stimulation, and for the baby to associate comfort and fullness with the breast, and keep the breast a happy place.

You might also pump several times throughout the day, save all that milk together in the fridge, and then warm it up and give 1 or 2 bottles a day of your own milk. Again, there is no right way, only your way. You can slice and dice all these different ways to feed your baby to come up with a routine that works for you and your family!

To protect supply long term it's also important to allow cluster feeding sessions as they come before moving on to offering a supplement—spend a few hours doing this before reaching for a bottle; or alternatively do power pumping every few days to mimic it. This means when your baby is having a growth spurt and wanting to feed every 5-30 minutes, you need to roll with it up to a point. If you don't get cluster sessions or power pump sessions you miss critical stimulation that builds and protects supply, long-term.

Power pumping is just like cluster feeding. There isn't a "right" way to do it, but there are suggestions on how to get it done. The most commonly suggested power-pump session involves pumping 20 minutes, taking a 10 minute break, pumping 10 minutes, taking one more 10 minute break, and then one final 10 minute pump session. Basically, it is back-to-back pump sessions in a short time period. You can also accomplish this by pumping a short 10-15 minutes session every hour for about 4-6 hours. Another way to accomplish power pumping is by squeezing in more short frequent pumps throughout the day so your total pumps per day are increased (for example pumping 10-12 times in one 24 hour period versus your normal 6-8). Even doing this part of the day gets the signals across—it tells the body, "Hey! I need more milk!"

When protecting lactation for combo fed babies, often nursing strikes come into play. This can cause accidental early weaning if not handled with care. Nursing strikes are when the baby is refusing to nurse. This can happen when they are startled during a feed, teething, start preferring bottle flow, or have a cold with congestion. Sometimes, the strike seems to come out of nowhere. Meet these strikes with the confidence that they will pass. Keep protecting supply by pumping and hand expressing, and offer the breast about 1-3 times daily in a low-stress way. Its best if baby is drowsy or asleep, and you try to get their instincts and reflexes to engage. A dark quiet room or co-bathing are both often successful environments to break a strike. Many babies who are in a nursing strike will still dream-feed, or nurse throughout the night. Paced feeding techniques help reduce the incidence of nursing strikes due to bottle preference.

Alternatively, a baby might exhibit a bottle strike. If they are over six months you can get them to take their fluids in sippy cups or straw cups. If they are under six months you can return to the basics like cup feeding, syringes, finger feeding, or at breast supplemental devices. Most strikes are short lived! It can help if the person giving the bottle is not the lactating parent, but yet makes the feed like a nursing session. This can mean draping a shirt that the lactating parent has worn over the caretaker, and feeding in the same spot to simulate a similar environment. There are tons of other techniques, and this is what IBCLC or feeding consults are for! Don't try to tough it out and go through these difficult times alone.

Its also important for protecting your supply long term to get mammary stimulation at peak prolactin time. Prolactin is on a circadian rhythm, as I mentioned before, it dips in the early evening. For most people it peaks in the late night to early morning, think 12 pm to 5 am. Getting stimulation between the peak hours sets the stage for your body to continue to keep making milk the next 24-48 hours. It is important to have some kind of stimulation to the breasts in these peak hours in order to keep your supply going.

In my book "Sleep Training the Breastfed Baby (or Not)" I explore in depth how to protect lactation when you start considering how you are going to balance lactation demands with sleep needs. When parents cut nighttime feeds it often leads to accidental early weaning, and causes babies to slow their weight gain because the milk supply the rest of the day drops, too.

Other generally helpful practices to help keep supply flowing when combo-feeding are often suggested for boosting supply, but they also work to protect it. These would be things like doing skin-to-skin with your baby regularly, spending time cuddling, baby-wearing, smelling your baby's head or worn clothes, and co-sleeping or breast-sleeping.

Pumping Successfully

Most combo-feeders employ pumping as a tool to help keep the lactation relationship going. This is especially true for lactating parents separated by work or custody arrangements. Some parents even prefer just to pump, or have a baby that can't successfully nurse. Whether pumping by choice or necessity, here are some tips to help.

The first step in pumping successfully is obtaining a pump. You should call your health care plan provider and work with them on which pumps are covered through your plan. Some providers will allow purchase when you are still pregnant, so give them a call in your third trimester. You can also consider purchasing pumps that are an upgrade or not covered on the plan. Usually, the most convenient cordless and tubeless versions are not covered (yet). The important aspects of a good pump are adequate suction and a proper fitting flange. It can be helpful to ask around in mom groups and read reviews when narrowing down your choices. The best pump for you is going to be a personalized choice, so you may need a consultation to get help choosing one.

Some general helpful things to look for in pump choice are these: a double electric pump that allows for dual stimulation (and thus more prolactin which usually means more milk), a vacuum strength of up to 250 mmHg, 2 modes to toggle through of stimulation and expression (to better mimic how babies eat), an electric cord and not just a battery, and at least 2 flange sizes with options to purchase other sizes.

Stimulation mode on a pump is a quicker cycle speed and weaker suction strength compared to expression mode; this mimics the suckling that babies do to get a letdown going. Expression is like a stronger slower gulping; like when babies take deep drinks during let downs.

You might have heard that cordless and wireless pumps are not great as a sole pump or for bringing in supply. While this may be true—if not having a cordless pump is going to keep you from pumping at all, then get one. More frequent sessions on a "lesser" pump is still better than skipped sessions because the pump isn't mobile. If mobility is a deal-breaker for you, try to find one that meets the above criteria and be sure to read a lot of reviews for figuring out the best one that is affordable for you. If you can swing it, get both a mobile and a more trusted wall-pump, so you can get at least some higher quality sessions in. You might find over time the "lesser" pump actually empties you better, as your body adjust to it.

I think even more importantly, getting the right flange fit is critical to pumping. Too small of flanges can cause friction blisters and prevent flow, both of which cause clogs. Too large of flanges pulls too much areola in and blocks ducts and causes bruising, both of which can cause clogs. Too small or too big can impede flow which means less milk. You want the fit to be "just right!" The nipple should move freely back and forth, without rubbing the sides and without too much areola being pulled in. Most pumps come with size 24-28 mm, and that's typically too large. For the best accuracy measure your nipples in millimeters, and add 2-3 mm to get the size you need. For wearable pumps the number you add is smaller, more like 0-2 mm. For example, if your nipple measures 15 mm, you would try to find a flange or flange insert that measures around 17-19 mm for a traditional pump and 15-17 mm for a wearable pump. Each nipple may be a different size, as few things in nature are perfectly symmetrical. When in doubt, first go with the tighter fit. After time goes on and we leave the pregnancy's hormonal influence, our nipples shrink. It is common to need to size-down flange size every few months the first year postpartum.

Other accessories that are helpful and might be covered by your HSA/FSA or insurance provider would be a milk cooler, ice packs, breast milk bags (reusable or plastic), extra sets of tubing, flanges, bottles, valves, membranes, a car adapter, and a pump bag to carry everything in! Gadgets like warming massagers might be covered too and can be very helpful for parents on the go who don't have the time to sit and hand massage, though they don't quite replace that hands-on stimulation. A hands-free pumping bra can be critical to making pumping convenient enough to maintain, and is sometimes covered as well.

Your pump parts that are soft like tubing and membranes will often need to be replaced every few months with regular use. They wear out and break down over time. Check with your pump manufacturer for how often and which parts need replaced regularly, and check with your HSA/FSA plan or insurance provider if those costs are reimbursable.

Another big question with pumping is when to start. This really depends on your plans and goals. If you know your baby will get bottles eventually, then you can start pumping right away. This leads me to explore further the myth that you should completely avoid pumping and bottles the first 6 weeks, at all costs. I believe this is a somewhat fair instruction for parents who will never be separated from their infant and do not plan to let others help or do not plan to return to work. Pumping and bottle feeding from the beginning will not ruin your breastfeeding relationship if balanced right. Furthermore, if this is what parenting choice you desire then you should be given information on how to most safely do this without sabotaging your over-all goals.

I think having this as a blanketed rule just creates room for confusion when new parents are told they need to pump within the first six weeks due to breastfeeding not going well. Having this blanket rule has caused parents to ignore the advice to start pumping when it was warranted, because this rule was drilled into their brain. You need to know that there is flexibility here, and while it is ideal to follow biological norms it is not going to derail your entire feeding journey if you have flexibility. Additionally, you may be instructed to start pumping to help get more milk to the baby if they are not feeding well, or to boost your supply.

Next, we will go over some issues that come up when pumping. One is milk color changes. This can be confusing and alarming to many parents, but it is not actually a problem in most cases. Your milk is not always white! It is first a golden yellow when it is colostrum in the end of pregnancy and the early days of nursing. It typically slowly adjusts to shades of white within 3 to 5 days postpartum. However, it can be many colors, usually based on your diet. A big batch of blueberries might tint it blue! Eat a lot of greens? Guess what? Green tinted milk! If it is pink it is likely from a bit of blood from an injury on your nipple, or a harmless growth in the breast, and is safe to feed. If it comes out of the breast white but then turns red after being out a while, this might be a harmful bacteria over-populating. It is never wrong when in doubt to seek professional guidance on if your milk is safe to feed or not.

The other perceived issue when looking at pumped milk is the fat content you are able to visualize. Sometimes, some of the fat separates out and gels at the top of the bottle, which looks like a large fat plug. Even if yours does not do this, there is likely still plenty of fat in it. The fat amount varies throughout the day and is generally higher in a more drained breast so more frequent feedings usually have higher fat content. You can eat more healthy fats to help improve the ratios of types of fats in the milk, but it is unlikely to increase the total fat content. Your baby needs the higher water volume of foremilk for hydration, and the higher concentration of fatty globules in the hindmilk for growth. Trust that your milk is made perfectly, the body has tens of thousands of years of practice built into its genetic coding. If you pump a large amount in one sitting be sure to mix it all together before separating it for feeds to ensure there is foremilk and hindmilk in each bottle.

Morning milk tends to have more volume, and less fat. Babies need to hydrate in the morning after going long stretches without drinking. Night milk tends to have less volume but more fat, and the higher fat in a full belly allows for greater satiety and longer stretches between feeds. Depending on the time of day the milk will have different levels of hormones and other particles to encourage baby to be awake or to sleep, such as tryptophan or melatonin. It is available in the milk to work with baby's natural hormone rhythms to encourage sleep and wake cycles; it is not enough to over-power the natural circadian patterns so do not worry too much about keeping track of what time you pumped your milk. Parents who do not track time pumped versus time fed have not been reporting a higher incidence of sleep issues in their infants, at least that I'm aware of. It does not hurt to track this and try to match these up, especially if you are struggling with getting to a normal sleep and wake pattern. It is not something to obsess over, just keep an eye on. A simple AM versus PM label would likely suffice for sorting, if you wanted to bother to sort that.

Pumped milk can also reveal a problem of having high lipase. Lipase is what helps break down the fats in the milk, and when there is a lot of it in pumped milk it can alter the smell and flavor. It can cause some babies to refuse pumped milk. It might taste or smell rancid, soapy, or metallic. It might change after a few hours, or only change after it has been frozen. This is easily remedied by scalding the milk right after it is pumped, which kills off some of the lipase. You would do well to test if you have high lipase before you start building a freezer stash in case you have a baby that refuses it.

The topic of pumped milk also inevitably begs the question of how it is different from fresh milk. Fresh milk is dynamic and changes to fit the baby's needs. Frozen milk may smell or taste different and have less white blood cells, less protein, less Vitamin C, and less antibacterial properties. The differences are negligible. It is still an excellent and preferred milk source compared to others! There is absolutely no harm in using pumped milk if handled with proper food safety measures.

Another invaluable form of expressing milk is called "hand expression." It is just what the name suggests—pumping out the milk using only your hands. There are excellent video tutorials on https://firstdroplets.com/abcs/ but it is a skill you have to practice to get good at. You can start practicing while pregnant. Hand expression and hands-on pumping are very valuable for getting an adequate supply. Don't forget: the hands-on approach should always be gentle.

Important Timeframes

Important timeframes to consider are these: the first month, 3-4 months, 6-9 months, and after 12 months. These are distinct time periods where things change up a bit. We will go into more detail here how you can navigate these times.

The first month is usually the most intense. It is the most critical time-frame for establishing a milk supply.   Babies start out eating very little amounts. How much they take in gradually goes up and up and up until they are about a month old. In the first 24 hours of life they take approximately 5-10 ml per feed. Throughout the first few days, every feeding they might take in around 20-30 ml (or 0.5 ounce). By the end of week one they have worked up to 45-60 mL per feed. It keeps gradually going up and by the time they reach a month, then they should take about 75-90 mL per feed (or 2.5-3 oz). This is about 1-1.5 ounces of milk per hour, once averaged out over a 24 hour period. This comes out to about 3 oz over about 8 feeds on average, so some babies take a bit more and some take a bit less. Twenty-five ounces or 750 ml over 24 hours is the average. Sometimes feed to feed the amount varies. Babies who take more might feed slightly less often. These numbers stay pretty stable from 1-6 months when solids are introduced.

It's important to note that most babies don't have the drive to only eat 6-8 times in a day, they often eat upwards of 12-16. Small frequent feeds are the biological design that works in tandem with the female body in order to bring in and build up milk supply. Feedings are often sporadic and sometimes very short. Especially the first two weeks, do not really count on your baby to behave like the books and guidelines say—expect random variation.

Knowing these numbers is helpful, but learning how to read your baby's body language is what helps guide your decisions around feeding. Even if it seems they are never satisfied, it is important to note that at times they actually are. To know if a baby is sometimes content, you will see their body give you clues. If they are truly never content, this might be a red flag and cause for concern. A content baby usually has open and relaxed hands, gets sleepy and drowsy at the breast after 10-15 minutes or more of nursing, their sucking starts to slow down, and they have good diaper output and weight gain. If they are nursing 30-45 minutes and coming off crying and upset, they may not be getting enough.

The reduction of baby's cluster feeding patterns coincides with our milk regulation hormonal patterns, first around 6 weeks and then again around 12 weeks. The erratic nursing pattern, or lack of a real pattern, is how the baby works with your body in tandem to continue to boost the supply the first 6 weeks. The cluster feeding and the sporadic nursing keep the breasts at a low volume compared to capacity, and this is what signals to the body to keep increasing the supply. This is why most lactation professionals discourage parents from putting a breastfed baby on a schedule. This is logistically challenging, as it makes planning around nursing tricky when there is lack of a schedule. As their schedule regulates or becomes more predictable so does the milk because your body starts to get the signal that the baby is more content.

If they never seem satisfied the first 4 to 6 weeks, it is because it is their job to act that way. This is part of the design of boosting the supply. Even bottle-fed babies will try to follow these instincts and cluster feed frequently the first 4-6 weeks. Their behavior, as such, is not the best or only indicator of adequate milk supply or transfer. The best indicators are diaper output and weight gain.

Around 3-4 months postpartum (or 12 weeks), as baby's needs are pretty stable, most lactating people experience supply regulation and sometimes this is a bit of a dip in the supply. Very few people see gains in amounts past this time frame. The breasts will stop feeling so full between feeds, and will generally have an over-all softer feel. Supply regulation worries a lot of first time parents, because they fear they are drying up.

When you are pumping more than nursing, you will see supply regulation, perceived as supply dips, at 3, 6, 9 and 12 months. As a pumping parent this will be more obvious, as the pumping output will decrease.

Pumping both mammae at the same time, or double pumping, helps you have a stronger hormonal response and will help get more milk out. Power pumping every few days will help keep supply boosted, as this mimics cluster feeding. Power pumping can be done several ways (as previously mentioned), but the general idea is to have a few pump sessions very close together, about 10-50 minutes apart, rather than 2-3 hours apart like routine pumping or feeding.

The timing of supply regulation also often coincides with needing to reduce flange size if you are pumping. The further postpartum you are, the more your nipples will shrink. Fit is important to maximizing breast drainage. You will want the flange to fit your nipple and have some clearance around it, but not pull too much areola in. If you are uncertain of fit, see your lactation consultant for help with sizing.

Around 3 months postpartum is also when many working mom's return to work, depending on where you live. I go into depth about challenges and changes around that in my book "Can I talk you out of breastfeeding?" if you want to go explore that particular information. The main things to know about combo feeding around this important time frame is covered pretty well here, but for those that like detail and in depth knowledge, that book is an excellent resource for lactating parents.

Around 6-9 months, babies really start getting into solids and a little bit into drinking water. This begins the process of "weaning," or slowly adding solids that eventually replace the milk as the main nutrition source. If you feed babies solids first thing at each feeding then secondarily offer the breastmilk or formula then babies will start to take more solids than breastmilk or formula, and this is undesirable the first year. Between 6 to 12 months it is ideal to breast or bottle feed first and then offer solids. After 1 year of age you can do either sequence.

The most recent literature suggests that sometime between 4 to 6 months most children are ready to start solids. I believe the body does not lie and their little bodies tell us when they are ready. Reading the body's readiness is better than just picking an arbitrary age of six months as the deciding factor. Six months was chosen as most baby's bodies are ready by then, but not all. Sleep regression at 4 months is often mistaken as a sign of readiness, but solid intake is not related to sleep habits. Babies' bodies signal they are ready for solids when they lose their tongue thrust reflex, they are able to sit up without assistance, and they have developed a pincher grasp.

Eating food between 6 and 12 months is for developmental milestones, practice with hand eye coordination, is an introduction to different flavors and textures, and provides some supplemental nutrition to their milk intake. They need practice with foods to be able to successfully eat well after age one. It also helps prevent the development of food allergies when you introduce foods before one year of age. The most recent evidence suggests we should introduce high allergen foods to babies before their first birthday.

This is also the time frame that you can start offering water. Babies should not get water before solids are started due to the danger it poses to their organs. Formula and breastmilk contain enough hydration and the right balance of electrolytes. This is also why properly mixing formula is so important; electrolyte imbalance due to too little or too much water is dangerous for babies. Small amounts of water with solids are okay, and might help prevent constipation. Several sources suggests around 4 to 8 ounces of water per day is safe between 6 to 12 months of age, so you can try offering 1-2 ounces each time you offer solids throughout the day. This will also help with practicing to use cups and straws, as the excitement of a new drink will encourage them to work towards using those items.

The only food you need to avoid the first year is honey, as their immune system is not ready to kill or destroy the botulism spores that might be present. This is true even of cooked honey, as heat does not destroy the spores. The only drink you need to avoid is any milk that is not formula or breastmilk. Dairy products can be introduced but other milks should not replace breastmilk or formula before they are 1 year old, as other milks do not have proper salt and fat content, which puts their kidneys and brain development at risk. It is also good practice to avoid sugary drinks like soda and juice, due to their connection to poor oral health and chronic disease development.

Around 12 months, a lot changes with lactation. Supply regulation shifts from being heavily hormone mediated and stimulation driven to being much more stable and available on demand. Solids can be a helpful tool to either help discourage or encourage nursing frequency, depending on your goals. Most toddlers nurse just a few times in 24 hours, rather than every few hours like babies. They no longer depend on it for their main sustenance, and it is a lovely compliment to their full and varied diet—rather than being their whole diet. This can relieve so much pressure on the lactating parent! Many people can stop pumping so frequently, or at least when separated from their baby, and just nurse on demand. Exclusive pumpers can cut out more pump sessions, yet keep making milk. The possibilities really open up by then, and you will have most things figured out.

Going through the relationship it's important to evaluate and then re-evaluate your routine regularly. Is it still working? What needs adjusted? Is it time I consulted an IBCLC? Remember, you don't have to take on these challenges alone.

Examples of Routines

So how do we combine all this together to make a feeding routine? Well, there is no simple answer to that. It will vary based on supply, preferences, and support. I will take the time to illustrate here some examples so you can brain-storm what routine might work best for you. A disclaimer to keep in mind: babies and boobs don't read books and your situation is not likely to look as neat and tidy as the examples I have laid out, so leave some room for nuance.

Example 1: The exclusive pumper

This dyad approaches feeding by deciding to pump and bottle feed right away. The lactating parent pumps every 4 hours from the beginning (knowing this is slightly less than ideal for a full supply), and the baby gets bottles on demand. The baby is paced-fed as often as they cue, and after ramping up the first month from newborn to infant levels takes around 2.5-5 oz each feed, anywhere from 8 to 12 times a day for the first few months. The parent's supply is robust in the morning, yielding 3-5 oz every session from 12 am to 12 pm, and then diminishes to 1.5-3 ounces when they pump between 12 pm and 12 am. This is fairly normal with prolactin circadian rhythms. Her baby eats 24-30 ounces every day and she pumps 20-24 ounces every day. The days she comes up short, she offers an a2 goat's milk formula bottle in the evening, keeping it the same size as the bottles he gets the rest of the day to avoid over-stretching his tummy. She is very anxious, and knowing the measurements of everything that goes in her baby helps her feel empowered and in control. She is able to pump 18 months, even with starting solids and some supply variation. She weans the baby's milk down as he takes on solids better, and eventually only gives him 5-10 ounces of her own milk in sippy cups split up over a whole day after he is 12 months old. This allows for her frozen pumped supply to stretch to last for him to get to have breastmilk for a total of 2 years.

Example 2: The at breast supplementer

This dyad has a parent with IGT and a micro-supply. She wants to provide whatever milk she can so she feeds every feeding at the breast, save one or two for a long stretch of 4-6 hours of sleep where her partner gives small bottles. She is able to attend consults with an IBCLC a few weeks in a row, and they weigh the feeds. They estimate together that baby is able to nurse out about 15-30 mL at each feeding, so they offer 2.5-3 ounces of supplemental standard formula in an at breast supplemental feeder. When Mom needs a break from time to time she skips a session and baby just gets a bottle. She maintains committed to 6 or more sessions at the breast every day, and most days it is around 8-10 sessions. She weighs the baby every week on a home scale and ramps up his supplement as needed based on him meeting weight gain goals, until they settle at 3-4 ounces each session. Around a year they wean off the SNS, but baby continues to comfort nurse at naptime, bedtime, and waking until he is 2 years old.

Example 3: The mixed bag

This dyad uses all the tools. When the lactating parent is most full, prolactin is highest, and milk is flowing—the baby goes to the breast. If baby ever seems unsatisfied, she finishes the feed at the breast with a large syringe giving half an ounce to an ounce. When her supply is lower in the evening they use the at breast supplemental nursing system (or SNS) for 1-2 feeds, adding 1-2 ounces into the SNS. When working with the IBCLC the baby's weighed feeds are always showing a 2-3 ounce transfer, which is great—but her baby sometimes needs a little more. She and her baby work off instincts and cues, and she just lets the baby take the lead. She commits to pumping every time a supplement is given the first 3 months, but after that—she lets it ride. The supply is what it is. She offers either pumped milk, or formula, whatever is handy. She pumps and bottle feeds the days she works, and then goes back to mostly breast when at home.

Example 4: The breast for dessert

This dyad has another parent with IGT. They work with an IBCLC to discover the baby is typically transferring about 1-2 ounces at every feeding. The baby is very frustrated by the slow flow, and does not like to take the breast before the bottle. Instead, the parent gives the baby 3 ounces of formula and then offers the breast for dessert. If the baby does not doze off to sleep and is still rooting for more milk then they offer another ounce of formula in the bottle. They decide on 3 ounces based on that baby's growth parameters are all on track with this amount. Unfortunately, its discovered through working with the pediatrician, that baby has a milk protein sensitivity, and mom has to go dairy free, and they have to switch to dairy free formula. Fortunately, this switch resolves all of baby's symptoms. Because parent and baby have breastfeeding as a positive and comforting association, the baby continues to nurse past a year even after they wean off bottles. They like to nurse after meals and before bedtime. This parent is eager to have another baby, and their supply dries out when they get pregnant again, so the baby stops nursing at that point around 16 months old.

Example 5: The top up

This dyad has a different plan, because her goal is not longevity. She has to return to the workforce at 6 months and does not want to have to pump while at work. She nurses on demand, and gives a top off when baby seems unsatisfied. She caps the top off to 1 ounce. She makes a full supply as far as she knows, but she likes using the formula for the flexibility. Her sticking to not giving more than 1 ounce top offs helps protect her supply. The morning feeds starting from around 3 AM to 10 AM, when she is most full, baby does not indicate he wants a top off. Her baby also gets a single 5 ounce bottle between 6 pm and 12 am, when she goes to get a long stretch of sleep and her partner takes over. Every evening she uses the pitcher method for her formula, and makes 10 ounces of formula and puts the pitcher in the fridge, pouring out what she needs as the day goes on. When she is within a month of returning to work she gradually increases the top offs by an ounce per feed every 3-5 days. Eventually her supply dwindles down in response. When she goes back to work baby is still nursing at night, but her daytime supply is so low that she is able to pump just once at lunch. She finds she is able to maintain that routine another 3 months, so they completely conclude nursing at 9 months when she dries up and baby is fully transitioned over to formula and solids. She feels really good about being able to provide breastmilk as long as she did, and felt the experience was relatively low stress.

Example 6: Every other feed

This lactating parent wants to give every other feed at the breast, and every other feed a bottle. She does this from the beginning. She meets with an IBCLC to get an estimate of feeding transfer and baby's needs. She nurses every 2-3 hours, and the baby gets a bottle every 2-3 hours. Standard formula seemed to make her baby constipated, so she switched to a hydrolyzed formula and the problem was resolved. If she ever gets to 4 hours without nursing and baby isn't hungry, she just pumps instead and freezes the milk for a "just in case" stash. She starts the process of weaning this routine at 1 year, so she can resume her IVF cycles to try for another baby. She is able to slowly transition off nursing and bottles as baby takes more and more solids and uses sippy cups, and she starts giving him goat milk to supplement his toddler milk needs. They fully weaned by 14 months as she went nice and slow to avoid clogs and mastitis.

Example 7: Pump all day, nurse all night

This parent has a robust night-time supply, but baby seems unsatisfied and unsettled at the breast during the day. From the beginning no supplementing is done at night. The baby and the parent breast-sleep and are happy to only nurse all night long. During the day, they utilize pumping and bottles. Since this needs to be done most days of the week when the lactating parent returns to work, they start with and keep it as the daily routine for consistency. Pump yield all day gets lower and lower as the day progresses. The first morning pump is usually 4-6 ounces, and then pumping every 3-4 hours after that they yield only another 1.5-3 ounces at each session. The baby takes 20-25 ounces throughout the day in 3-5 ounce bottles. The pump yield is only 10-15 ounces. For what is lacked, the parent uses a friend's donated milk to make up the difference. When solids are introduced the gap between what is pumped and what is taken via bottle narrows. Daily pump output is 10-12 ounces but bottles are reduced to a daily intake of 15-20 ounces. The friend continued to donate. This dyad goes on to nurse 3 years, and the parents were able to wean off bottles between 12 and 16 months.

Example 8: The triple feeder

This parent's goal is to maximize supply and longevity of the nursing relationship. She has a history of low supply with other children. Every feeding except one in the evening, she breastfeeds and then pumps while offering a bottle. During the evening she takes a 4-6 hour break to rest, and her partner gives a bottle or two on demand. Through the night she parallel pumps, so she pumps while she nurses. What is pumped is given to the baby by her partner so she can get back to sleep. They maintain this routine for about 3 months, at which time the lactating parent drops their pumping entirely when home with their infant. At 3 months they do a combination of nursing, pumping when at work, and bottle feeding. The only exception is that she continues to triple feed her first morning feed of the day between 5 to 7 am when she wakes for the day, in order to maximize yield from when her prolactin is very high in the morning.

If the baby nurses prior to a bottle they then take 1.5-2 ounces of formula or pumped milk. If the baby gets a bottle only (while the lactating parent is unavailable or at work), she takes 4-5 ounces. Sometimes through the night the baby will just nurse and go back to sleep, and not root for a bottle after. When solids start, the baby does not consistently finish her bottles and usually takes 0.5-1 ounce, but sometimes in the evening still takes a full 2 ounce supplement. Because the baby takes such small supplemental amounts they use pre-made formula that comes in 2 ounce jars, all year. They are able to maintain this routine for the rest of the first year, at which time they drop bottles but continue to nurse. This dyad goes on to nurse 2-3 times a day until the child is 5 years old.

Final Thoughts

Being a good parent starts with caring how well you parent. I believe one of our many jobs as parents is to advocate for our children. We do that in part by educating ourselves as much as possible on what an optimal situation might look like and what potential complications might look like. We take the information we learn and push for what we have concluded is best, given our circumstances. This looks quite different for each family, and for each individual child. The options and opinions are many, so you will have to figure out what works for you.

With our first basic task of feeding we can read books and take prenatal classes and meet with IBCLCs. However, I will invite you to remember that you are so much more than a milk maker. A parent provides nourishment in many forms. Parents provide so much more than food to help their babies thrive. You will provide for your baby's basic needs which will teach your baby about love and trust.

It will not matter much when they are adults if they got formula, but it will influence their health if you spend their early formative months stressed. If you want to breastfeed: feed the baby, protect your supply, and keep the breast a happy place. Do those three things and then seek help! Use the formula! Just know how to protect your lactation relationship. Seek help early, and often. It is critical to get an evaluation and plan from a professional who knows you and your baby's medical history.

Truthfully, with everything the modern lactating parent faces it seems like we are set up to fail. That is why the USA national rates of initiating are around 79-95% depending on region, but the continuation drops to 20-50% by 6 months. Statistically--most of us are formula fed and go on to formula feed, at least partially. Many cultural messages around breastfeeding make it hard to trust our body. Our culture and our laws do not protect the sacred relationship that is breastfeeding. I hope our culture continues to shift back towards supporting the norms of breastfeeding, and the parent-infant dyad's relationship. This does not mean that in doing so we will stop using formula or stigmatize it's use. I hope we continue to see not only the rates of initiation of breastfeeding rise, but the continuation of the breastfeeding relationship at higher rates and for longer stretches of time. I want combo-feeding to be a tool to help reach those goals, and formula can play a huge part in that. I hope that arming more parents with this knowledge that I have imparted through this book will contribute to this change.

I implore you not to go into a breastfeeding relationship with hard rules or expectations. Being flexible is what will make you resilient. It will also help preserve your sanity. Be ready for steep and staggering personal growth. When you are pushed to your limits, you will learn your limits. Leave space in your breastfeeding relationship and leave space in your parenting to grieve that which will not come to pass, no matter how much you will it. Managing your expectations for what is realistic and possible will in turn help manage your mental health. Hope for the best and prepare for the worst. Leave space to celebrate what is working and what is enjoyable about the experience. There is always room for the joy and gratitude of what is, and it is also okay to be sad and grieve for what is not. Make room for it all.

∞∞∞

If you would like more information on all the challenges that can come up when breastfeeding and lactation, please check out my other book "Can I Talk You Out of

Breastfeeding?" It is a tongue in cheek title, challenging you to ask yourself if you would still want to breastfeed if you were given all the ins-and-outs of how hard it can be.

If you want more information on balancing lactation with sleep needs, please check out my book "Sleep Training the Breastfed Baby (or Not)." This teaches you how to protect lactation and balance your sleep needs, whether or not you sleep train.

If you enjoyed this book and learned from it, please leave me a review through the platform that you purchased the book from and recommend it to your friends. I am also always open to polite debate and constructive criticism, as I am always seeking to learn.

Resources

You should have a healthcare team set up to help you face potential challenges. Start with meeting with an IBCLC. Choose a breastfeeding supportive pediatrician. Ask them questions about what ways they support breastfeeding, and make sure their ideals match yours. Bring in a speech and language pathologist, and myofunctional therapist and body workers like massage therapists, chiropractors and cranial sacral therapists as needed for feeding difficulties. Have an idea of who you would talk to or go see if you feel you needed emotional or mental health support. Ask around your local community for recommendations of these specialists. Build your healthcare village.

Remember that everyone you know is a resource. Your support circle needs to grow, and you should be the one to grow it. Do not wait for people to volunteer, tell them how they can help. When people do offer to help, tell them something specific you want. If someone is willing to do something for you, let them.

Do not forget the amazing resource of technology that we have as modern parents. You can get many free apps on your phone to track feedings, diapers, sleep, measurements, and milestones. You can utilize social media and search engines for many things, as long as you also consult your professional team. Social media can also be very beneficial to combatting isolation and loneliness, as it can connect you with other parents. You can send pictures and video-chat with family if you do not want to have them over, or if they live too far to visit. You can also attend online classes, do online prenatal consults, attend online support groups, and watch how-to videos of many of the hands-on skills you will need like pumping, swaddling, and burping.

You are also a powerful resource unto yourself. You can do a lot to prepare. Go to a prenatal consult. Take the parenting and breastfeeding classes, read the books, do the meal-prep, freeze some padsicles, do the mental and emotional work. Manage your own expectations. Take responsibility for yourself by asking for help and setting boundaries. Give yourself grace, compassion, and patience. Trust your instincts. Seek help early and often.

Find an IBCLC

You need support from a local or virtual IBCLC. When you see a lactation consultant, like myself, I suggest a prenatal lactation assessment to review your risk factors and take steps specific to your risks to maximize your supply before pregnancy, during, and immediately postpartum. They can help in the early weeks and up until weaning, even if that is well into childhood.

Even without some of these problems breastfeeding is generally challenging. Becoming a new parent is challenging. Lean into your community and reach out for help. Do not wait until there is a problem; see an IBCLC before pregnancy, during, and after. Let them monitor your progress in those fragile early weeks. Let them help you troubleshoot, perfect, and optimize your breastfeeding experience.

I am available virtually, find me on Instagram @sophia.felder.fnp.ibclc and post education content regularly. Local appointments may be available and might be covered by insurance if you are on the Olympic Peninsula in Washington State. I occasionally open my schedule for private consults online, when time allows.

Utilize your lactation benefits through insurance

The Affordable Healthcare Act, signed into law in 2010, ensures that more females in the United States have access to coverage for lactation support and pumping equipment. As of the writing of this book in 2020, this is still in effect. Health insurance plans, outside of grandfathered plans and certain state Medicaid plans, must provide breastfeeding support and equipment for the duration of breastfeeding, and some help is available during pregnancy. This means you are able to get a prenatal lactation consult, and possibly get your pump before baby comes. The pump provided might be a rental, manual, or electric. Some require birth of the baby before they will issue the pump. It should be up to you and your provider which option is best for you, and they can write a prescription to be filled by a medical supply company. Some plans cover other equipment like bags or valve replacements, or they are at least FSA/HSA (Flexible Spending or Healthcare Spending accounts) eligible. Much of the breastfeeding and pumping paraphernalia is covered under FSA/HSA spending, so always check before you purchase or check if you are eligible for reimbursement. The equipment offered may require partial cost-sharing if you choose to upgrade, but a no-cost option should also be available. The lactation support might need to be with an in-network provider, require prior-authorization, or referral. Lactation services are considered preventative medicine, as lactation is a biological expectation, and you should not have any co-pays, payments toward deductible, or co-insurance fees. If you see an OB/GYN, CNM, pediatrician, or FNP (like me) who is also an IBCLC you might be covered under preventative medicine as well, and this may not count towards using the lactation consult benefit. This is important to know if your plan places a limit on number of visits per year. This is information you want to clarify while you are still pregnant so you can plan ahead and have help lined up for when you inevitably need it.

Here is a helpful toolkit to help you understand your rights under this law, and suggestions to hold your plan accountable if they are not meeting the standards set forth by the law. www.nwlc.org/sites/default/files/pdfs/final_nwlcbreastfeedingtoolkit2014_edit.pdf

Find an oral tether/tongue tie provider

If you suspect your child has oral tethers it is best to find a "preferred provider" with a reputation for doing thorough work. Follow up with finding stretches and exercises for oral tethers; you can start these even before a revision. This is where you will want to involve your healthcare village. Visit www.tt-lt-support-network.com/

There are also many Facebook support groups, usually separated by state, where you can get feedback from other parents who have seen providers in your area. They also typically share how their recovery process was, and other associated therapists, consultants, and bodyworkers in the area that aided in their post-procedure recovery and functional optimization.

Infant Risk

A top resource for what medication is safe during pregnancy and breastfeeding. They have a website, app called MommyMeds, book, and hotline. Visit www.infantrisk.com/

Jack Newman, M.D. Breastfeeding Medicine Specialist; Newman's website is an excellent resource for breastfeeding information. Visit www.breastfeedinginc.ca/

"Safe Infant Sleep" a book by James J McKenna, Ph.D. Visit cosleeping.nd.edu/ to learn more about the Mother-Baby Behavioral Sleep Lab at the University of Notre Dame.

PPD/PPA Resources

Postpartum Support International: Visit www.postpartum.net/

Warm Line (non-emergent phone support): 1 800 944 4773

Postpartum Support International offers phone support, online chat support, online support meetings and local resources. Online support meetings are held weekly for both moms and dads. Information is available at this site in both English and Spanish.

Text HOME to 741741 if you need immediate assistance you can find help 24 hours a day, 7 days a week and have a cell phone and are in the United States. Their website explains their services. Visit www.crisistextline.org/text-us/

Call the National Suicide Prevention Hotline at 1800 273 8255, which is also available 24/7

Domestic Abuse Resources

National Domestic Violence Hotline, which has a website with education and resources, as well as a chat feature, in addition to their hotline phone number. Visit www.thehotline.org

When you go to the website you will be prompted with this warning: "Internet usage can be monitored and is impossible to erase completely. If you are concerned your internet usage might be monitored, call us at 1 800 799 SAFE (7233). Learn more about digital security and remember to clear your browser history after visiting this website. Click the "X" or "Escape" button at any time to leave TheHotline.org immediately."

Kellymom website, which is a breastfeeding and parenting guide; visit Kellymom.com

Substance Abuse and Mental Health Services Administration

Hotline number is 1-800-662-4357

Visit their website at www.samhsa.gov/find-help/national-helpline